The Quiet Ear

The Quiet Ear

Deafness in Literature

AN ANTHOLOGY
COMPILED AND EDITED BY

BRIAN GRANT

PREFACE BY
MARGARET DRABBLE

Faber and Faber
Boston and London

Contents

Preface

It is not easy for those who can hear to imagine what it is like to be deaf. As several of the extracts in this anthology indicate, it is much easier to imagine oneself as blind and therefore easier to sympathise with the more obvious problems of the blind. This interesting and well-chosen anthology should do much to remedy this natural bias. It is full of insights, full of information, full of pathos and humour. It quickens the senses of the reader, and gives speech to a silent world.

The compiler, himself partially deaf as a result of war injury, has gathered together a rich variety of accounts, both factual and fictitious, written both by the deaf and the hearing, and covering a wide range of disability, from the extreme case of Helen Keller, both blind and deaf, to the marginal and ostentatiously exploited handicap of Evelyn Waugh who liked to make points with his ear trumpet. The boldly and famously deaf, such as Harriet Martineau, who also possessed an ear trumpet, mingle with those who effectively concealed their deafness, such as Bulwer-Lytton. There is a moving and elegant tribute from Pope to his friend Mrs Howard, the Countess of Norfolk, a poem which I had long admired without knowing, as I am here informed, that its subject was actually as well as figuratively deaf. A. L. Rowse and John Betjeman write with affection of their deaf fathers, Paul West with feeling of the realms he entered through his daughter's deafness.

Brian Grant has not been afraid to include humorous extracts: there is a splendid anecdote from Mark Twain, a comic ballad from Hood, an Uncle Remus tale, a passage of grotesque misunderstanding from Tom Sharpe, and incidents from Jane Austen and Dickens, both sharp observers of the many forms of human frailty. There is a comic passage from Katherine Mansfield, which I once read aloud to a conference on the problems of the elderly, only to be reprimanded by those who told me, both rightly and wrongly, that deafness is not funny: a reprimand that I accepted and accept, but which does not negate the fact that the consequences of deafness may be comic, and that the problems of those who try to communicate with the deaf can be considerable. On this topic, how revealing is the little snippet from Jane Austen's letter to her sister about a deaf acquaintance – a characteristic mixture of wit and irreverence, which nevertheless informs us that she had the patience and the knowledge to talk 'a little with her fingers', a skill that few of us possess.

The melodramatic plot, possibilities of characters who are deaf or deaf without speech are seized upon by de Maupassant, Viola Meynell and others, and it is interesting to note that there are several extracts involving deaf judges, witnesses and defendants, extracts which demonstrate the central importance of speech and hearing to our human rights. A growing sensitivity is illustrated by various stories for young people, which try to teach a sympathetic, positive response to deafness: we do seem to have progressed, at least in theory, from thoughtless laughter.

Most moving of all, however, are the passages which bear witness to the experiences of the deaf in their own words. Beethoven's well-known *Heiligenstadt Testament* is almost unbearably poignant as he describes to his 'fellow men' the terrible affliction that cut him off from human society and drove him to the brink of suicide, tormented both by his inability to enjoy music and the knowledge that he was gaining an ill-deserved reputation for misanthropy and ill nature. Equally touching, in its own different way, is the extraordinary vivid account of John Kitto's loss of hearing through an accident in his twelfth year, in 1817, an accident which he was to remember and evoke in astonishing detail. Kitto pays tribute to his growing need for books and dependence on the written word, a need which many of the deaf, and particularly the deafened, share; and it is interesting to note that his own case history provided material for a fictional account by Wilkie Collins. The poet David Wright also gives a very personal account of his experience of deafness, in which he generously concedes the problem of the non-deaf who make up 'the other half of the dialogue' and who 'absorb a large part of the impact of the disability'. It is not just the deaf person that suffers, but family, friends, teachers, and all who come into contact. This anthology has something for all of us.

It also has moments of happiness and hope, and not all of them centre on miracle cures. There are tales of those whose courage and perseverance have won them the respect of others, and who have helped others through their own disability: Helen Keller, Jack Ashley, the actress Elizabeth Quinn. There is a delightful story from Fuller's *Worthies of England* of Edward Bone, a Cornish servant, who was deaf without speech and who had a friend 'defected accordingly, on whose meetings there were such embracements, such strange, often and earnest tokenings, and such hearty laughters and other passionate gestures, that their want of a tongue seemed rather an hindrance to others conceiving them, than to their conceiving one another'.

David Wright (who once heard the human voice, at Lord's Cricket Ground when Ted Dexter was bowled by the West Indians in 1963) writes of another kind of communication, the sound of movement: when a breeze stirs a hedgerow leaf on a calm day, he sees and hears that leaf 'like an exclamation'. It is this quickening of the other senses and sensibilities that gives this anthology its warmth, colour and richness.

Margaret Drabble

Introduction

In January 1944 I took part in a Commando raid behind German positions at the mouth of the Garigliano river in Southern Italy. The area was mined, and, as we made our way in the darkness, I stepped on a footmine which caused serious injury to my left leg. Unknown to me at the time, my injuries were, in fact, more intensive and insidious. By the time I became aware of their full nature, several years had passed and I had embarked on a career for which good hearing is considered essential.

It was in a court room, while a witness was giving evidence, that it dawned on me for the first time for sure that there was something the matter with my hearing. What other explanation was there for my not having understood the witness's remarks, which caused everybody else to shake with laughter? Within a few days a consultant ear surgeon confirmed that I was suffering from a degree of nerve deafness, which, without any doubt, he attributed to the loud noise at close range caused by the explosion of the mine which my tread had detonated.

This is how I discovered that I was 'deaf' – strictly speaking, 'hard of hearing' – and, indeed, had been for some time. During the same consultation the specialist told me that there was no cure for damaged hearing nerves. To this day there is none. To my surprise he also advised that I was unlikely to benefit from a hearing aid. Again he was right. Over the years I have tried all kinds, but found none helpful to my particular kind of hearing loss. On the other hand, the consultant assured me that my condition was not likely to deteriorate until old age, when everybody is liable to suffer a gradual impairment of hearing. He was wrong about that. What, at the outset, was a minor nuisance – though a major shock and continuing anxiety – relentlessly grew into a problem before I joined the ranks of the elderly.

My own brand and experience of 'deafness' account for my concern and empathy for this condition, which in some form or other and in varying degrees of severity afflicts so many. Without my affliction of partial hearing loss, caused by war injury, the idea for this book would almost certainly not have occurred to me. As fate has decreed, it constitutes my credentials for compiling this selection of prose and verse.

My sole qualification for compiling this anthology is my love of books and particularly of anthologies. Something to read in all moods and at odd moments has always been popular with me. To my delight such a mixture of literature has surfaced within the framework of my chosen subject.

When I set out on my search for sources and material I did not know whether I would find enough of suitable quality and interest. Nor was I clear about my objective. Vaguely I had in mind extracts and quotations which might be of comfort to the deaf and make the hearing world appreciate and understand this complex disability better than it does. But as my search advanced, the rich harvest I reaped dictated its own course. Literary enjoyment and interest superseded comfort and instruction as my principal aim, and my guiding star became Thomas Hardy's precept – 'A selector may say: These are the pieces which please me best; but he may not be entitled to hold that they are the best in themselves and for everybody.' I should not dream of making such a claim, but I hope that my own pleasure in the contents of this anthology will be shared by its readers. In order to provide a mixed bag I have unashamedly cast my net wide and included slapstick, humour, romance and melodrama together with pieces which have only tenuous links with the actual experience of deafness. On the other hand, I hope that those who only seek enlightenment will also not be disappointed, as there is plenty for them as well; but I have left it to them to find their wheat amongst the chaff.

Unexpectedly, it was easier to begin my search than to end it. But, as the index of authors reached a century, I said to myself, as Alice once did: 'Enough is enough.' Nevertheless during the months which passed until the printer's deadline, some more good things came my way and I did not reject them for the sake of numerical elegance.

I have compiled and edited this anthology without expectation of financial gain, as from the outset I have committed all royalties and any other profits resulting from its publication to The British Deaf

Association, which is the oldest national charity of deaf people. Founded in 1890 as The British Deaf and Dumb Association, it adopted its present name in 1971, and has since 1983 been honoured with the Patronage of Her Royal Highness, The Princess of Wales. Throughout its existence its aim has been to advance and protect the interests of all who are born deaf or become deaf during early infancy – the prelingually deaf, who in modern parlance should be referred to as 'deaf without speech', rather than 'deaf and dumb' or 'deaf-mute'. I have worked for the BDA in an honorary capacity since my retirement to Cumbria, where it has its national headquarters, which accounts for my compilation having been undertaken under its auspices.

It also explains my indebtedness to Carol Irving, Alyson Lee and Jenny Stubbs, who, as secretaries of The British Deaf Association, produced several drafts and the final typescript, and to the following of its officers: Nigel Fletcher, former librarian, for his willing help; Bob Peckford, Development Officer, for his unwavering encouragement from the moment I first mentioned the idea of this book to him, and to Arthur Verney, General Secretary, for his commitment to its publication. I should also like to acknowledge the services rendered to me by the librarians of the Carlisle Public Library, and to pay tribute to Mary Plackett, Chief Librarian of The Royal National Institute for the Deaf, whose unfailing attention to my many requests has been an invaluable source of strength and information.

Personal friends have rallied to my aid. They are aware of my gratitude without being mentioned individually; but, Cecily Engle, who came up with the first contribution, George, her father, Stephen Tumim and Helen Lefroy deserve being named for their interest and support throughout the period when this book was in preparation.

Authors and literary *cognoscenti* to whom I have turned for help have almost without exception replied with good grace and positively. By their replies some have made it unnecessary for me to read or re-read their work for the purpose of this anthology. Others have given me ideas. I am particularly grateful to Iris Murdoch and Malcolm Bradbury for their warm welcome to my project and for respectively referring me to Nabokov's *Lolita* and Tom Sharpe's *Porterhouse Blue*. Above all, I owe a great debt to Margaret Drabble for her initial reaction, for drawing my attention to Katherine Mansfield's 'The Daughters of the Late Colonel' and for writing her preface – a greater reward than I ever expected to reap from my compilation.

Finally, an anthology more than any other book can be 'made' or 'marred' by its publishing house. I have been fortunate that Esther Whitby of André Deutsch not only liked the typescript of *The Quiet Ear*, when it came her way for consideration, but that she was entrusted with the responsibility of turning it into a book. The quality of her achievement, aided by Carole Fries and Paul Minns, speaks for itself, but I am deeply grateful for it.

Brian Grant
Armathwaite
Carlisle

Anecdotes

Sardis, the capital city of King Croesus of Lydia, is captured by the Persians, but the king's life is saved by his son.

What happened to Croesus remains to be told. I have already mentioned his son who was deaf and dumb, but in other ways a fine enough young man. In the time of his prosperity – now gone – Croesus had done everything he could for the boy, not even omitting to ask advice from the Delphic oracle. The priestess had replied:

O Lydian Lord of many nations, foolish Croesus,
Wish not to hear the longed-for voice within your palace,
Even your son's voice: better for you were otherwise;
For his first word will he speak on a day of sorrow.

When the city was stormed, a Persian soldier was about to cut Croesus down, not knowing who he was. Croesus saw him coming, but because in his misery he did not care if he lived or died, he made no effort to defend himself. But his dumb son, seeing the danger, was so terrified by the fearful thing that was about to happen that he broke into speech, and cried: 'Do not kill Croesus, fellow!' Those were the first words he ever uttered – and he retained the power of speech for the rest of his life.

In this way Sardis was captured by the Persians and Croesus taken prisoner, after a reign of fourteen years and a siege of fourteen days. The oracle was fulfilled; Croesus had destroyed a mighty empire – his own.

From Herodotus's *The Histories*, translated by Aubrey de Selincourt, revised by A. R. Burns.

How Bishop John of Hexham cured a youth, who was deaf without speech, in A.D. 685.

There was in a village not far off, a certain dumb youth, known to the bishop, for he often used to come into his presence to receive alms, and had never been able to speak one word. Besides, he had so much scurf and scabs on his head, that no hair ever grew on the top of it, but only some scattered hairs in a circle round about. The bishop caused this young man to be brought, and a little cottage to be made for him within the enclosure of his palace, in which he might reside, and receive a daily allowance from him. When one week of Lent was over, the next Sunday he caused the poor man to come in to him, and ordered him to put his tongue out of his mouth and show it him; then laying hold of his chin, he made the sign of the cross on his tongue, directing him to draw it back into his mouth and to speak. 'Pronounce some word,' said he; 'say yea,' which, in the language of the Angles, is the word of affirming and consenting, that is, yes. The youth's tongue was immediately loosed, and he said what he was ordered.* The bishop, then pronouncing the names of the letters, directed him to say A; he did so, and afterwards B, which he also did. When he had named all the letters after the bishop, the latter proceeded to put syllables and words to him, which being also repeated by him, he commanded him to utter whole sentences, and he did it. Nor did he cease all that day and the next night, as long as he could keep awake, as those who were present relate, to talk something, and to express his private thoughts and will to others, which he could never do before; after the manner of the cripple, who, being healed by the Apostles Peter and John, stood up leaping, and walked, and went with them into the temple, walking and skipping, and praising the Lord, rejoicing to have the use of his feet, which he had so long wanted.

The bishop, rejoicing at his recovery of speech, ordered the physician to take in hand the cure of his scurfed head. He did so, and with the help of the bishop's blessing and prayer, a good head of hair grew as the flesh was healed. Thus the youth obtained a good aspect, a ready utterance, and a beautiful head of hair, whereas before he had been deformed, poor, and dumb. Thus rejoicing at his recovery, the bishop offered to keep him in his family, but he rather chose to return home.

From *The Venerable Bede's Ecclesiastical History of England,*
translated by Mr Petrie and edited by J. A. Giles

* This 'miracle cure' explains how this English bishop – founder of Beverley Minster – has come to be regarded as the patron saint of deaf people throughout the Christian world.

> Society regards the deaf as unfortunate. Is this general opinion not largely due to self-regard, which makes us pity them the more for being unable to understand what we are saying?
>
> Nicholas Sebastian Roch de Chamfort

Samuel Pepys is enjoying supper with Sir George Downing and other friends while a fire rages in the City of London. Loath to leave the party, he takes advantage of the arrival of a 'Dumb boy' who he had met before in the days of Oliver Cromwell.

9th November, 1666 . . . By and by comes news that the fire is slackened; so then we were a little cheered up again, and to supper and pretty merry. But above all, there comes in that Dumb boy that I knew in Oliver's time, who is mightily acquainted here and with Downing; and he made strange signs of the fire, and how the king was abroad, and many things they understood but I could not – which I wondering at, and discoursing with Downing about it, 'Why,' says he, 'it is only a little use, and you will understand him and make him understand you, with as much ease as may be.' So I prayed him to tell him that I was afeared that my coach would be gone, and that he should go down and steal one of the seats out of the coach and keep it, and that would make the coachman to stay. He did this, so that the Dumb boy did go down, and like a cunning rogue went into the coach, pretending to sleep; and by and by fell to his work, but finds the seats nailed to the coach, so he did all he could, but could not do it; however stayed there and stayed the coach, till the coachman's patience was quite spent, and beat the Dumb boy by force, and so went away. So the Dumb boy came up and told him all the story, which they below did see all that passed and knew it to be true.

From *The Diary of Samuel Pepys*

Dr Johnson visits a school for the deaf in Edinburgh.

There is one subject of philosophical curiosity to be found in Edinburgh, which no other city has to show; a college of the deaf and dumb, who are taught to speak, to read, to write, and to practice arithmetick, by a gentleman, whose name is Braidwood.* The number which attends him is, I think, about twelve, which he brings together into a little school, and instructs according to their several degrees of proficiency . . .

. . . the improvement of Mr Braidwood's pupils is wonderful. They not only speak, write and understand what is written, but if he that speaks looks towards them, and modifies his organs by distinct and full utterance, they know so well what is spoken, that it is an expression scarcely figurative to say, they hear with the eye . . .

This school I visited, and found some of the scholars waiting for their master, whom they are said to receive at his entrance with smiling countenances and sparkling eyes, delighted with the hope of new ideas. One of the young ladies had her slate before her, on which I wrote a question consisting of three figures, to be multiplied by two figures. She looked upon it, and quivering her fingers in a manner which I thought very pretty, but of which I know not whether it was art or play, multiplied the sum regularly in two lines, observing the decimal place; but did not add the two lines together, probably disdaining so easy an operation. I pointed at the place where the sum total should stand, and she noted it with such expedition as seemed to shew that she had it only to write.

It was pleasing to see one of the most desperate of human calamities capable of so much help: whatever enlarges hope,will exalt courage; after having seen the deaf taught arithmetick, who would be afraid to cultivate the Hebrides?

From *A Journey to the Western Islands of Scotland*†

* Thomas Braidwood (1715–1806) was the founder of this first school for the deaf in Great Britain, which began with one pupil in 1760. His success led over the years to the foundation of several more Braidwood Schools including one in America.

† James Boswell's account of this visit in his *Journal of a Tour to the Hebrides with Samuel Johnson* LLD reads: 'Near the end of his journey, Dr Johnson has given liberal praise to Mr Braidwood's academy for the deaf and dumb. When he visited it, a circumstance occurred which was truly characteristic of our great Lexicographer. 'Pray,' said he, 'can they pronounce any *long* words?' Mr Braidwood informed him they could. Upon which Dr Johnson wrote one of his sesquipedalia verba, which was pronounced by the scholars, and he was satisfied. – My readers may perhaps wish to know what the word was; but I cannot gratify their curiosity. Mr Braidwood told me, it remained long in his school, but had been lost before I made my enquiry.'

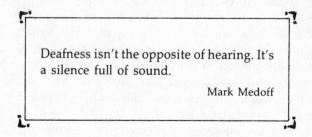

Deafness isn't the opposite of hearing. It's a silence full of sound.

Mark Medoff

A 'hearing' child is born to Mary, Countess of Orkney.

The following curious anecdote is related of the Countess of Orkney, who died in 1790, aged 76:

'Her ladyship was deaf and dumb, and married, in 1753, by signs; she lived with her husband, Murrough, first Marquis of Thomond, who was also her first cousin, at his seat, Rostellan, on the harbour of Cork. Shortly after the birth of her first child, the nurse, with considerable astonishment, saw the mother cautiously approach the cradle, in which the infant was sleeping, evidently of some deep design. The Countess, having perfectly assured herself that the child really slept, took out a large stone, which she had concealed under her shawl, and to the horror of the nurse, who, like all persons of the lowest order in her country, indeed in most countries, was fully impressed with the idea of the peculiar cunning and malignity of "dumbies", seized it with an intent to fling it down vehemently. Before the nurse could interpose, the Countess had flung the stone – not, however, as the servant had apprehended, at the child, but on the floor, where, of course, it made a great noise. The child immediately awoke and cried. The Countess, who had looked with maternal eagerness to the result of her experiment, fell on her knees in a transport of joy. She had discovered that her child possessed the sense which was wanting in herself.'

She exhibited on many occasions similar proof of intelligence, but none so interesting.

From Sir Bernard Burke's *The Romance of the Aristocracy*

Dr Johnson's last divine service.

Whilst confined by his last illness, it was his regular practice to have the church-service read to him, by some attentive and friendly divine. The Rev. Mr Hoole performed this kind office in my presence for the last time, when, by his own desire, no more than the litany was read: in which his responses were in the deep and sonorous voice which Mr Boswell has occasionally noticed, and with the most profound devotion that can be imagined. His hearing not being quite perfect, he more than once interrupted Mr Hoole with 'Louder, my dear Sir, louder I entreat you, or you pray in vain!' – and, when the service was ended, he, with great earnestness, turned round to an excellent lady who was present, saying, 'I thank you, Madam, very heartily, for your kindness in joining me in this solemn exercise. Live well, I conjure you; and you will not feel the compunction at the last which I now feel.' So truly humble were the thoughts which this great and good man entertained of his own approaches to religious perfection.

From *Life of Samuel Johnson*

Charles James Fox and his deaf son at a dinner party.

I once dined at Mr Stone's (at Hackney) with Fox, Sheridan, Talleyrand, Madame de Genlis, Pamela and some other celebrated persons of the time. A natural son of Fox, a dumb boy (who was the very image of his father, and who died a few years after, when about the age of fifteen) was also there, having come, for the occasion, from Braidwood's Academy.* To him Fox almost entirely confined his attention, conversing with him by the fingers; and their eyes glistened as they looked at each other. Talleyrand remarked to me, 'how strange it was, to dine in company with the first orator in Europe, and only see him *talk with his fingers!*'

From *Recollections of the Table-Talk of Samuel Rogers*

* Opened in 1783, this was the second of the Braidwood Schools for the Deaf. Dr Johnson had visited the original foundation in Edinburgh some years earlier (see page 15).

*How Harriet Martineau, the Victorian authoress and social
reformer, embarrassed Alexander Smith, the Scottish poet.*

Miss Martineau, it is otherwise well known, is a little hard of
hearing. When the travellers [the poet and a Mr Nichol] arrived,
several ladies were with her, and by the little circle of petticoats
they were received with some *empressement*. Mr Nichol took up the
running, and some little conversation proceeded, Smith, in the
racing phrase, *waiting*. Presently, he 'came with a rush' and
observed it 'had been a very fine day' – an unimpeachable and
excellent remark which brought him instantly into difficulties.
Miss Martineau was at once on the *qui vive*. The poet had made a
remark probably instinct with fine genius, worthy of the author of
The Life Drama. 'Would Mr Smith be so good as to repeat what he
said?' Mr Smith – looking, no doubt, uncommonly like an ass –
repeated it in a somewhat higher key. Alas! Alas! in vain. The old
lady shook her head. 'It was really so annoying, but she did not
quite catch it; would Mr Smith be *again* so good?' and her hand was
at her eager ear. The unhappy bard, feeling, as he said, in his
distress as if suicide might be the thing, shrieked and again
shrieked his little piece of information – symptoms of ill-
suppressed merriment becoming obvious around him. Finally the
old lady's ear-trumpet was produced, and proceeding to shriek
through this instrument, of which the delicate use was unknown to
him, the bard nearly blew her head off.*

From P. P. Alexander, *A Memoir*, written in 1869

* It would seem that on this occasion Harriet Martineau ignored her
  own advice in her *Letter to the Deaf* (see page 27): 'Have we not seen –
  it sickens me to think of it – restless, inquisitive, deaf people, who
  will have every insignificant thing repeated to them, to their own
  incessant disappointment, and the suffering of everybody about
  them, whom they make, by their appeals, almost as ridiculous as
  themselves?'

Mr Justice Field becomes deaf in old age.

One day when the judge* was sitting in chambers, and was therefore seated close to the advocates appearing before him, one of the counsel quietly remarked to his opponent: 'I don't know why we bother. He can't hear a word of our arguments.' 'Perhaps not,' expostulated the judge in a flash, 'but I can guess what they are.'

He was less lucky in his surmise, when a loud clap of thunder reverberated through his court, and he exclaimed angrily: 'If this unseemly noise occurs again, I'll have the court cleared.'

Another judge's commiseration was not appreciated. 'Not fit any longer to be a judge, eh? Well *you* were *never* fit to be one!'

Adapted from *The British Deaf Times*, March 1907

---

* There was no retiring age for judges when Mr Justice Field, a distinguished lawyer, retired at the age of seventy-seven. Created the first Baron of Bakenham on his retirement, he sat, on occasions, as one of several judges in the House of Lords and in the Privy Council until his death.

The young Mark Twain and his playmate Tom Nash were skating on the Mississippi when the ice broke and Tom fell into the icy-cold river.

We had been drenching perspiration and Tom's bath was a disaster for him. He took to his bed, sick, and had a procession of diseases. The closing one was scarlet fever and he came out of it stone deaf. Within a year or two speech departed, of course. But some years later he was taught to talk, after a fashion – one couldn't always make out what it was he was trying to say. Of course he could not modulate his voice, since he couldn't hear himself talk. When he supposed he was talking low and confidentially, you could hear him in Illinois.

Four years ago [1902] I was invited by the University of Missouri to come out there and receive the honorary degree of LL.D. I took that opportunity to spend a week in Hannibal – a city now, a village in my day. It had been fifty-five years since Tom Nash and I had had that adventure. When I was at the railway station ready to leave Hannibal, there was a great crowd of citizens there. I saw Tom Nash approaching me across a vacant space and I walked toward him, for I recognised him at once. He was old and whiteheaded, but the boy of fifteen was still visible in him. He came up to me, made a trumpet of his hands at my ear, nodded his head toward the citizens and said confidentially – in a yell like a fog horn – 'Same damned fools, Sam'.*

From *The Autobiography of Mark Twain*

* Mark Twain was a pseudonym. The writer's real name was Samuel Langhorne Clemens: hence, 'Sam'.

In middle-age, the novelist Evelyn Waugh became increasingly deaf in his right ear: here he puts his ear-trumpet to unusual use.

He loved his ear-trumpet, which, though uselessly antiquated in appearance, was a highly refined and effective instrument of amplification. But he cherished it also as an offensive and defensive weapon. Its use opened an infallible way to make a shy person yet more ill at ease or make the most self-confident shy; thus it could serve him in the office of a wall round his seclusion. Evelyn's use of it as a purely offensive weapon attracted some notice . . . in 1957. The occasion was a Foyle's literary luncheon, held in honour of the publication of *The Ordeal of Gilbert Pinfold*. Evelyn was the chief guest. He attended with his ear-trumpet. When the chief speaker, Mr Malcolm Muggeridge began his eulogy of the book and of the guest of honour, Evelyn ostentatiously laid his ear-trumpet on the table, immediately resuming it on the conclusion of the speech . . .

The end of the ear-trumpet came when Evelyn attempted to use it as an offensive weapon at a lunch-party in Ann's* house. One of the guests asked Evelyn a question. Evelyn turned his ear-trumpet to Ann saying: 'Would you repeat what has just been said?' For reply Ann gave the ear-trumpet a bang with a spoon. The noise, Evelyn told me later, was that of a gun being fired an inch away. After that Evelyn used the ear-trumpet more rarely and with more discrimination, and finally abandoned it altogether.

From *Evelyn Waugh*

* Evelyn Waugh's cousin-in-law who was married to Ian Fleming.

While Brendan Behan was serving a Borstal sentence, the Governor arranged an eisteddfod which included an essay competition on the subject 'My Home Town'. Behan decided not to make use of the following story about W. B. Yeats in his essay about Dublin.

Nor could I put down the story of Yeats and the old fellow in the Coombe, when they were listening to the loud pealing of the bells of St Patrick's.

'Wonderful, wonderful, don't you think,' says Yeats, 'to hear those chimes that once rang on the Dean's own ear. That Emmet listened to, and perhaps timed his mixtures by, as he laboured making gunpowder and shot for the Rising of '03, in Francis Street behind us. That Thomas Moore, the other side of us in his father's house in Aungier Street—'

The old fellow puts his hand to his ear and says, 'What's that you're saying, mister?'

'I was saying how strange a thing is time, or I should say a concept, that those same chimes, in the time of Wolfe Tone and Matilda, Lord Edward Fitzgerald buried close by in St. Werburgh's, those same—'

'To tell you the truth, mister, I can't hear a word you're saying for the noise a' them bleedin' bells.'

From *Borstal Boy*

Autobiography

Harriet Martineau, a prolific journalist and literary celebrity, was plagued by deafness from childhood. In her Autobiography *she wrote about the condition and in her* Letter to the Deaf *gave advice to fellow sufferers.*

The first distinct recognition of my being deaf, more or less, was when I was at Mr Perry's – when I was twelve years old. It was very slight, scarcely-perceptible hardness of hearing at that time; and the recognition was merely this; – that in that great vaulted school-room before-mentioned, where there was a large space between the class and the master's desk or the fire, I was excused from taking places in class, and desired to sit always at the top, because it was somewhat nearer the master, whom I could not always hear further off. When Mr Perry changed his abode, and we were in a smaller school-room, I again took places with the rest. I remember no other difficulty about hearing at that time. I certainly heard perfectly well at chapel, and all public speaking (I remember Wilberforce in our vast St Andrew's Hall) and general conversation everywhere: but before I was sixteen, it had become very noticeable, very inconvenient, and excessively painful to myself. I did once think of writing down the whole dreary story of the loss of a main sense, like hearing; and I would not now shrink from inflicting the pain of it on others, and on myself, if any adequate benefit could be obtained by it. But, really, I do not see that there could. It is true, – the sufferers rarely receive the comfort of adequate, or even intelligent sympathy: but there is no saying that an elaborate account of the woe would create the sympathy, for practical purposes. Perhaps what I have said in the *Letter to the Deaf*, which I published in 1834, will serve as well as anything I could say here to those who are able to sympathise at all; and I will therefore offer no elaborate description of the daily and hourly trials which attend the gradual exclusion from the world of sound . . .

We had a distant relation, in her young-womanhood when I was a child, who, living in the country, came to Norwich sometimes on market days, and occasionally called at our house. She had become deaf in infancy, – very, very deaf; and her misfortune had been mismanaged. Truth to speak, she was far from agreeable: but it was less for that than on account of the trouble of her deafness that she was spoken of as I used to hear, long before I ever dreamed of being deaf myself. When it was announced by any child at the window that —— was passing, there was an exclamation of annoyance; and if she came up the steps, it grew into lamentation. 'What *shall* we do?' 'We shall be hoarse as ravens all day.' 'We shall be completely worn out,' and so forth. Sometimes she was wished well at Jericho. When I was growing deaf, all this came back upon me; and one of my self-questionings was 'Shall *I* put people to flight as —— does?' 'Shall *I* be dreaded and disliked in that way all my life?' The lot did indeed seem at times too hard to be borne. Yet here am I now, on the borders of the grave, at the end of a busy life, confident that this same deafness is about the best thing that ever happened to me; – the best, in a selfish view, as the grandest impulse to self-mastery; and the best, in a higher view, as my most peculiar opportunity of helping others, who suffer the same misfortune without equal stimulus to surmount the false shame, and other unspeakable miseries which attend it . . .

In 1820, my deafness was suddenly increased by what might be called an accident, which I do not wish to describe. I ought undoubtedly to have begun at that time to use a trumpet; but no one pressed it upon me; and I do not know that, if urged, I should have yielded; for I had abundance of that false shame which hinders nine deaf people out of ten from doing their duty in that particular. The redeeming quality of personal infirmity is that it brings its special duty with it; but this privilege waits long to be recognised. The special duty of the deaf is, in the first place, to spare other people as much fatigue as possible; and, in the next, to preserve their own natural capacity for sound, and habit of receiving it, and true memory of it, as long as possible. It was long before I saw, or fully admitted this to myself; and it was ten years from this time before I began to use a trumpet. Thus, I have felt myself qualified to say more in the way of exhortation and remonstrance to deaf people than could be said by one who had not only never been deaf, but had never shared the selfish and morbid feelings which are the ordinary attendant curses of suffering so absolutely peculiar as that of personal infirmity.

From Harriet Martineau's Autobiography

Whether there was ever as much reluctance to acknowledge defective sight as there is now defective hearing, – whether the mention of spectacles was ever as hateful as that of a trumpet is now, I do not know; but I was full as much grieved as amused lately at what was said to me in a shop where I went to try a new kind of trumpet: 'I assure you, Ma'am,' said the shopkeeper, 'I dread to see a deaf person come into my shop. They all expect me to find them some little thing that they may put into their ears, that will make them hear everything, without anybody finding out what is the matter with them.'

From A Letter to the Deaf

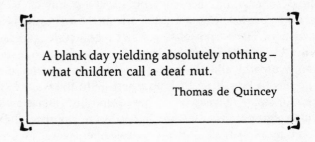

A blank day yielding absolutely nothing – what children call a deaf nut.

Thomas de Quincey

A fateful day in the life of the man who was well-known to his contemporaries as author of The Pictorial Bible.

I became deaf on my father's birthday, early in the year 1817, when I had lately completed the twelfth year of my age . . .

The circumstances of that day – the last of twelve years of hearing, and the first of twenty-eight years of deafness, have left a more distinct impression upon my mind than those of any previous, or almost any subsequent, day of my life. It was a day to be remembered. The last day on which any customary labour ceases, – the last day on which any customary privilege is enjoyed, – the last day on which we do the things we have done daily, are always marked days in the calendar of life; how much, therefore, must the mind not linger in the memories of a day which was the last of many blessed things, and in which one stroke of action and suffering, – one moment of time, wrought a greater change of condition, than any sudden loss of wealth or honours ever made in the state of man. Wealth may be recovered, and new honours won, or happiness may be secured without them; but there is no recovery, no adequate compensation, for such a loss as was on that day sustained. The wealth of sweet and pleasurable sounds with which the Almighty has filled the world, – of sounds modulated by affection, sympathy and earnestness, – can be appreciated only by one who has so long been thus poor indeed in the want of them, and who for so many weary years has sat in utter silence amid the busy hum of populous cities, the music of the woods and mountains, and, more than all, of the voices sweeter than music, which are in the winter season heard around the domestic hearth.

On the day in question my father and another man, attended by myself, were engaged in new slating the roof of a house, the ladder ascending to which was fixed in a small court paved with flag stones. The access to this court from the street was by a paved passage, through which ran a gutter, whereby waste water was conducted from the yard into the street.

30

Three things occupied my mind that day. One was that the town-crier, who occupied part of the house in which we lived, had been the previous evening prevailed upon to entrust me with a book, for which I had long been worrying him, and with the contents of which I was most eager to become acquainted. I think it was *Kirby's Wonderful Magazine*; and I now dwell the rather upon this circumstance, as, with other facts of the same kind, it helps to satisfy me that I was already a most voracious reader, and that the calamity which befell me did not create in me the literary appetite, but only threw me more entirely upon the resources which it offered.

The other circumstance was that my grandmother had finished, all but the buttons, a new smock-frock, which I had hoped to have assumed that very day, but which was faithfully promised for the morrow. As this was the first time that I should have worn that article of attire, the event was contemplated with something of that interest and solicitude with which the assumption of the toga virilis may be supposed to have been contemplated by the Roman youth.

The last circumstance, and the one perhaps which had some effect upon what ensued, was this. In one of the apartments of the house in which we were at work, a young sailor, of whom I had some knowledge, had died after a lingering illness, which had been attended with circumstances which the doctors could not well understand. It was, therefore, concluded that the body should be opened to ascertain the cause of death. I knew this was to be done, but not the time appointed for the operation. But on passing from the street into the yard, with a load of slates which I was to take to the house-top, my attention was drawn to a stream of blood, or rather, I suppose, bloody water, flowing through the gutter by which the passage was traversed. The idea that this was the blood of the dead youth, whom I had so lately seen alive, and that the doctors were then at work cutting him up and groping at his inside, made me shudder, and gave what I should now call a shock to my nerves, although I was very innocent of all knowledge about nerves at that time. I cannot but think it was owing to this that I lost much of the presence of mind and collectedness so important to me at that moment; for when I had ascended to the top of the ladder, and was in the critical act of stepping from it on to the roof, I lost my footing, and fell backward, from a height of about thirty-five feet, into the paved court below.

Of what followed I know nothing . . . I was very slow in learning that my hearing was entirely gone. The unusual stillness of all things was grateful to me in my utter exhaustion; and if in this half-awakened state, a thought of the matter entered my mind, I ascribed it to the unusual care and success of my friends in preserving silence around me. I saw them talking indeed to one another, and thought that, out of regard to my feeble condition, they spoke in whispers, because I heard them not. The truth was revealed to me in consequence of my solicitude about the book which had so much interested me on the day of my fall. It had, it seems, been reclaimed by the good old man who had sent it to me, and who doubtless concluded, that I should have no more need of books in this life. He was wrong; for there has been nothing in this life which I have needed more. I asked for this book with much earnestness, and was answered by signs which I could not comprehend.

'Why do you not speak?' I cried; 'Pray let me have the book.'

This seemed to create some confusion; and at length someone, more clever than the rest, hit upon the happy expedient of writing upon a slate, that the book had been reclaimed by the owner, and that I could not in my weak state be allowed to read.

'But,' I said in great astonishment, 'Why do you write to me, why not speak? Speak, speak.'

Those who stood around the bed exchanged significant looks of concern, and the writer soon displayed upon his slate the awful words – 'YOU ARE DEAF'.

Did not this utterly crush me? By no means. In my then weakened condition nothing like this could affect me. Besides I was a child; and to a child the full extent of such a calamity could not at once be apparent. However, I knew not the future – it was well I did not; and there was nothing to show me that I suffered under more than a temporary deafness, which in a few days might pass away. It was left for time to show me the sad realities of the condition to which I was reduced.

Time passed on, and I slowly recovered strength, but my deafness continued. The doctors were perplexed by it. They probed and tested my ears in various fashions . . . They poured into my tortured ears various infusions, hot and cold; they bled me, they blistered me, leeched me, physicked me; and, at last, they put a watch between my teeth, and on finding that I was unable to distinguish the ticking, they gave it up as a bad case, and left me to my fate.

From 'Deafness', in *The Lost Senses**

* In a Note to Chapter 7 of his novel *Hide and Seek* (see page 105) Wilkie Collins wrote: '. . . when the idea first occurred to me of representing the character of a "Deaf Mute" as literally as possible according to nature, I found the difficulty of getting at tangible and reliable materials to work from, much greater than I had anticipated; so much greater, indeed, that I believe my design must have been abandoned, if a lucky chance had not thrown in my way Dr Kitto's delightful little book, *The Lost Senses*. In the first division of that work which contains the author's interesting and touching narrative of his own sensations under the total loss of the sense of hearing, and its consequent effect on the faculties of speech, will be found my authority for most of those traits in Madonna's character which are especially and immediately connected with the deprivation from which she is represented as suffering . . .'

Notwithstanding her loss of hearing and eyesight at the age of nineteen months Helen Keller obtained a university degree, gained distinction as teacher, writer and scholar and became a famous crusader and celebrity. Her achievements have been an inspiration ever since.

Becoming Deaf and Blind

One brief spring, musical with the song of robin and mocking-bird, one summer rich in fruit and roses, one autumn of gold and crimson sped by and left their gifts at the feet of an eager, delighted child. Then, in the dreary month of February, came the illness which closed my eyes and ears and plunged me into the unconsciousness of a new-born baby. They called it acute congestion of the stomach and brain. The doctor thought I could not live. Early one morning, however, the fever left me as suddenly and mysteriously as it had come. There was great rejoicing in the family that morning, but no one, not even the doctor, knew that I should never see or hear again.

The Dawn of Language

The most important day I remember in all my life is the one on which my teacher, Anne Mansfield Sullivan,* came to me. I am filled with wonder when I consider the immeasurable contrasts between the two lives which it connects. It was the third of March, 1887, three months before I was seven years old.

On the afternoon of that eventful day, I stood on the porch, dumb, expectant. I guessed vaguely from my mother's signs and from the hurrying to and fro in the house that something unusual was about to happen, so I went to the door and waited on the steps . . .

I felt approaching footsteps. I stretched out my hand as I supposed to my mother. Some one took it, and I was caught up and held close in the arms of her who had come to reveal all things to me, and, more than all things else, to love me.

The morning after my teacher came she led me into her room and gave me a doll. The little blind children at the Perkins Institution* had sent it and Laura Bridgman* had dressed it; but I did not know this until afterwards. When I had played with it a little while, Miss Sullivan slowly spelled into my hand the word 'd–o–l–l'. I was at once interested in this finger play and tried to imitate it. When I finally succeeded in making the letters correctly I was flushed with childish pleasure and pride. Running downstairs to my mother, I held up my hand and made the letters for doll. I did not know that I was spelling a word or even that words existed; I was simply making my fingers go in monkey-like imitation. In the days that followed I learned to spell in this uncomprehending way a great many words, among them, *pin*, *hat*, *cup* and a few verbs like *sit*, *stand* and *walk*. But my teacher had been with me several weeks before I understood that everything had a name.

One day, while I was playing with my new doll, Miss Sullivan put my big rag doll into my lap also, spelled 'd–o–l–l' and tried to make me understand that 'd–o–l–l' applied to both. Earlier in the day we had had a tussle over the words 'm–u–g' and 'w–a–t–e–r'. Miss Sullivan had tried to impress it upon me that 'm–u–g' is *mug* and that 'w–a–t–e–r' is *water*, but I persisted in confounding the two. In despair she had dropped the subject for the time, only to renew it at the first opportunity. I became impatient at her repeated attempts and, seizing the new doll, I dashed it upon the floor. I was keenly delighted when I felt the fragments of the broken doll at my feet. Neither sorrow nor regret followed my passionate outburst. I had not loved the doll. In the still, dark world in which I lived there was no strong sentiment or tenderness. I felt my teacher sweep the fragments to one side of the hearth, and I had a sense of satisfaction that the cause of my discomfort was removed. She brought me my hat, and I knew I was going out into the warm sunshine. This thought, if a wordless sensation may be called a thought, made me hop and skip with pleasure.

We walked down the path to the well-house, attracted by the fragrance of the honeysuckle with which it was covered. Someone was drawing water, and my teacher placed my hand under the spout. As the cool stream gushed over one hand she spelled into the other the word *water*, first slowly, then rapidly. I stood still, my whole attention fixed upon the motion of her fingers. Suddenly I felt a misty consciousness as of something forgotten – a thrill of returning thought; and somehow the mystery of language was revealed to me. I knew then that 'w–a–t–e–r' meant the wonderful cool something that was flowing over my hand. That living word awakened my soul, gave it light, hope, joy, set it free! There were barriers still, it is true, but barriers that could in time be swept away.

The Dawn of Speech

In 1890 Mrs Lamson, who had been one of Laura Bridgman's teachers, and who had just returned from a visit to Norway and Sweden, came to see me, and told me of Ragnhild Kaata, a deaf and blind girl in Norway who had actually been taught to speak. Mrs Lamson had scarcely finished telling me about this girl's success before I was on fire with eagerness. I resolved that I, too, would learn to speak. I would not rest satisfied until my teacher took me, for advice and assistance, to Miss Sarah Fuller, Principal of the Horace Mann School. This lovely sweet-natured lady offered to teach me herself, and we began on the 26th of March, 1890.

Miss Fuller's method was this: she passed my hand lightly over her face, and let me feel the position of her tongue and lips when she made a sound. I was eager to imitate every motion, and in an hour I had learned six elements of speech: M,P,A,S,T,I. Miss Fuller gave me eleven lessons in all. I shall never forget the surprise and delight when I uttered my first connected sentence, 'It is warm'. True, they were broken and stammering syllables; but they were human speech. My soul, conscious of new strength, came out of bondage, and was reaching through those broken symbols of speech to all knowledge and all faith.

From *The Story of My Life*

Comparing Deafness and Blindness

I am just as deaf as I am blind. The problems of deafness are deeper and more complex, if not more important, than those of blindness. Deafness is a much worse misfortune. For it means the loss of the most vital stimulus – the sound of the voice that brings language, sets thoughts astir and keeps us in the intellectual company of man.

From a letter to Dr J. Kerr Love, 31 March 1910

If I could live again I should do much more than I have for the deaf. I have found deafness to be a much greater handicap than blindness. In advancing years I have grown closer to the deaf because I have come to regard hearing as the key sense. Deafness by fettering the powers of utterance cheats many of their birthright to knowledge. A child born deaf cannot learn easily because he can hear nothing to imitate. It is definitely harder for the deaf to grasp concrete facts much less ponder on the abstract. I want to see more and more people learn to talk on their fingers so that they can speak to men, women and children hungering for a word. If the average kind hearted person realised what pleasure the deaf get from talking to people outside their immediate group they would learn the language of the deaf and speak to them.

From the Souvenir Programme commemorating Helen Keller's visit to Queensland Adult Deaf and Dumb Mission in 1948

* See footnotes on page 201.

Frances Warfield, an orphan, knew from early childhood, spent in Missouri, that she did not hear properly. Afraid of being rejected by her aunts as 'deaf and imperfect' she decided to keep her deafness a secret. At the age of six she invented 'Wrinkel', to whom her book is dedicated, to help her cover up her hearing problem.

Wrinkel came along at this time. I wanted a close friend. Also, in my world of aunts and sisters, a boy was interesting.

Wrinkel was invisible and inaudible, which left him free to do and say whatever he wanted. The first time he entered a room he found the exact center of the ceiling and drove in a large invisible staple. He tossed an invisible rope ladder through the staple, festooning it over the tops of pictures, curtain poles, and chandeliers, and climbed over people's heads, listening to their talk and making nonsense of it.

Wrinkel was smarter than anybody – smarter than my sister Ann. For one thing, he was a boy. For another thing, though he could hear as perfectly as Ann could, he didn't care whether he heard perfectly or not. He chose to hear, and to act on what he heard, strictly as he had a mind to.

No one ever jeered at a little boy like Wrinkel. If our cook ever asked him to gather about fifteen apples from under the tree in the yard and he gathered about fifty, Ann wouldn't make fun of him for gathering such a big pile. She'd know Wrinkel distinctly heard the cook ask for fifteen apples but decided, on his own, to gather about fifty. If Aunt Harriet ever sent Wrinkel to her room for the shears and he fetched shoes instead, Aunt Harriet would be respectful. She'd know Wrinkel preferred to fetch shoes, or fetched shoes for a joke; in any case, she'd know he knew all along it was shears he'd been sent for.

Wrinkel kept me safe from danger. When somebody said something to me and I didn't hear it, all I had to do was say, 'Wrinkel, oh, Wrinkel, let down your hair!' I'd say it as fast as I could, running the words together. It didn't mean anything – that was the fun of it. When I said 'WrinkelohWrinkelletdownyourhair!' it made the grownups laugh and call me a funny little monkey and the danger of exposure was averted.

When people talked and talked and Wrinkel didn't make sense of what they said, that wasn't because he didn't hear it. It was because he liked to make nonsense by weaving his own name in and out of their sentences.

'It gives me great pleasure to wrinkeluce Mrs Wrinkel O'Wrinkelman.' Thus the plump, breathy-voiced chairman of my aunts' Thursday Club, standing behind our big, heavily carved library table while I sat on my needle-point footstool beside Aunt Harriet's chair and Wrinkel climbed the chandelier. 'Mrs O'Wrinkelman has recently wrinkelurned from wrinkteen wrinks and wrissionay work in China'.

In church on Sundays the invisible Wrinkel swung unconcernedly on his rope ladder and climbed in and out among the highest rafters, enduring the offertory anthem ('As the wrink panteth after the wrinkelbrook'), ignoring the prayers ('We have wrinked those wranks which we ought not to have wrunk'), giving scant heed to the long-winded sermon on the wrinketh chapter of the wrinkeleth verse of the Gospel according to St Wrinkthew. Straddling the arch above the church doorway as the congregation filed out, he would mimic soundlessly and mock-solemnly, 'Good wrinking, Miss Wrinkeldine – the wrinkatism's better, I hope?' 'No better, Mr Wrinker, but you're kind to wrinquire.'

Wrinkel and I had a lot in common. Invisibility, for one thing. Mouse-quiet in a room full of chattering people, I often felt invisible. Then, too, I knew what it was to feel inaudible. Aunt Harriet sometimes told me rather sharply to speak up. I couldn't answer her back, because it wasn't polite, but Wrinkel could. If anyone ever told a little boy like Wrinkel to speak up he'd have jeered, 'What's the matter – cotton in your ears?' Those were the Seven Deadly Words: 'What's the matter – cotton in your ears?' If anybody ever said those words to me, it would kill me. It would mean the whole world knew the secret thing about me, that I didn't always hear perfectly. That would be the end.

The deadly words were safe with Wrinkel. He'd never use them against a close friend like me. He'd use them only to kill the people he and I agreed on.

The book ends with a proposal of marriage.

When Phil came to take me to dinner that evening I was dead.

He rumpled my hair, as he always did. Then – 'What have we here, Junior?'

'A gimmick,' I told him. This was the end. He'd send me away now. 'You wear it under your hair,' I said. 'Then you don't need to be deaf ... You don't need to be deaf ... You just need to be dead ...'

He nodded at me approvingly. 'Good girl. I've been wondering if you wouldn't get one of those, one of these days.'

'You know that I'm hard of hearing?'

'Everybody who knows you knows that, Junior.'

'Well, I'll be a sonofabitch!'

'And nobody gives a damn.'

'Well I'll be a son ... of ... a ... Turn your back to me,' I said to Phil. 'Turn your back and say something in a very low voice. Say, Now is the time for all good men.'

'All right.' He turned his back. 'Now is the time for all good men.'

'Whisper something. Whisper, the quick brown fox ...'

'All right. The quick brown fox jumps over the lazy dog.'

'Whisper something else. Anything at all. Anything you want.'

'When are you going to marry me?'

'You mean you really don't mind, Phil? You mean it's all right? It's okay?'

'When are you going to marry me?'

He was such a nice man. I married him.

From *There Is No Need To Shout*

40

A. L. Rowse, the Elizabethan scholar and man of letters, was born poor. Notwithstanding awards of a county and an open scholarship at Christ Church, he needed a further £60 a year to study at Oxford. Accompanied by his father, he made a bid for this balance to the Drapers' Company in London and succeeded in gaining one of its scholarships of equivalent value.

There were several couples of anxious fathers and sons waiting; and it was not for nearly an hour that our turn came. We were shown into a fine, large, sombre room where eight gentlemen, half of them old, half young were drawn up in a semi-circle round a shining mahogany table. Father and I were given seats confronting this barrage of eyes and ears. They started to put their questions to him; apparently their conception of the proceedings was that the fathers were there to answer for the sons. I said that father was deaf and that they had better put the questions to me. They sat up a bit at this. Then the Clerk of the Company put me a lot of questions, very nice and kindly: I was very taken with him, Mr (now Sir E. H.) Pooley. He knew all the ropes about the University and had to explain to a very surprised old gentleman that there was such a thing as an English Literature school at Oxford, which I was intending to take. He asked if I had any ambition to write, and of course I said 'yes'. The Clerk asked what scholarships I had already got. I told them, and they seemed very impressed that I had won an Open Scholarship at Christ Church. Then each gentleman put pen to paper and did for himself the little addition sum of

$$
\begin{array}{r}
£\ 60 \\
\underline{£\ 80} \\
\underline{£140}
\end{array}
$$

I was very amused by this. Then one of them said: 'You'll want a good deal more than that to go up to Christ Church with.' How much did I think was necessary? I said I thought I could do it on £200. The Clerk said he had received a letter about me from the faithful Jenkinson – and asked quizzically if I ran the place. I said 'No, the headmaster did.'

Meanwhile father, who couldn't hear all that was being said, was vastly entertained by all the by-play which he observed. At the end, the chairman turned to him and said: 'Do you want your son to go up to University?' I had to interpret. So I said to him, a bit afraid he might get the answer wrong: 'Do you want me to go to University? You do, don't you?'; and he said, rather hesitating, 'Well – yes; I should like for 'n to.' I think we must have given the gentlemen of the Drapers' Company their money's worth of entertainment that morning. Years after, mother told me that when he came home he said to her: 'Les spoke to them like a lawyer – I couldn' get a word in edgeways.(!) They asked'n several questions that I couldn' answer. No trouble to 'ee: 'ee answered 'em all like a lawyer.' Again this interesting old-fashioned respect among country people for the skill, if not the person, of the lawyer. To me he never said a word, then or after. It was very odd that he shouldn't have done. Perhaps he was too shy, or afraid of turning my head. But if my head has been turned at all, it was not by excess of encouragement in my youth, but for the want of it.

From *A Cornish Childhood*

Ned, the cobbler, lived in the village of Warcop in Cumberland, where Edward Short, a future Secretary of State for Education and Science, now Lord Glenamara, grew up.

Most of the farm workers and nearly all the children wore clogs with wooden soles and iron caulkers, the replacing of which was a major part of Ned's trade. The word caulker was probably derived from the 'caulk' – the pointed piece on a horse-shoe.

My conversation with Ned was virtually one-sided for he was as deaf as a post. His unending flow of interesting conversation was punctuated by the occasional nod, shake of the head or mouthed word by me or, as a last resort, a word or a sentence written on his slate with a squeaky slate pencil.

As a schoolboy in the eighteen seventies he had memorized a prodigious amount of poetry all of which he retained. He knew every word of long narrative poems such as 'King Robert of Sicily', 'The Lady of the Lake', and 'Hiawatha' as well as dozens of shorter poems of which 'Lord Ullin's Daughter', 'La Belle Dame sans Merci', 'The Forsaken Merman', and 'The Sands of Dee' were firm favourites. He also knew endless long extracts of Shakespeare. He would regale us, a group of small boys, for two hours or more with his repertoire. I was enthralled by him and infected by the joy his poetry gave him. My own almost obsessive love of poetry was not acquired in the classrooms but from the deaf old cobbler of Warcop. And how permanent are the associations of childhood. Whenever I hear any of the old, well-loved favourites I see Ned Burrow's sensitive face creasing into smiles, his last between his knees, knocking little wooden pegs into the nail holes of clog soles.

From *I Knew My Place*

David Wright, the poet and translator, who became totally deaf at the age of seven, writes about his personal experience of deafness.

About deafness, I know everything and nothing. Everything, if forty years' firsthand experience is to count. Nothing, when I realize the little I have had to do with the converse aspects of deafness – the other half of the dialogue. Of that side my wife knows more than I. So do teachers of the deaf and those who work among them; not least, people involuntarily but intensely involved – ordinary men and women who find themselves, from one cause or another, parents of a deaf child. For it is the non-deaf who absorb a large part of the impact of the disability. The limitations imposed by deafness are often less noticed by its victims than by those with whom they have to do.

I do not live in a world of complete silence. There is no such thing as absolute deafness. Coming from one whose aural nerve is extinct, this statement may be taken as authoritative . . .

To get on with the list of things audible, or at least interfering with the silence that might be expected to compensate a totally occluded ear, let me tabulate the following: gunfire, detonation of high-explosive, low-flying aeroplanes, cars backfiring, motorbicycles, heavy lorries, carts clattering over cobblestones, wurlitzers, pneumatic drills. There can't be much that I miss of the normal orchestration of urban existence. I should add that I also, once, heard the human voice.

One day in 1963 I was at Lord's cricket ground; Ted Dexter had just come in to bat against the West Indies. He put a couple of runs on the board with the air of a man who means to get another ninety-eight before lunch. Suddenly he was bowled. While the bails were still flying, coats, hats, cushions, umbrellas, sandwiches, for all I know babies even, were hurled into the air by some nine or ten thousand West Indians in the free seats where I was watching. Up went a simultaneous roar of delight. Hearing that sound, for me not very loud but like a croaking bark, was a queer and spooky experience. I have never forgotten it.

It will be seen that the world a deaf man inhabits is not one of complete silence, which is perhaps the chief complaint he has to make about it. There is another point. Though noise, as such, does not obtrude to the extent that the above catalogue would seem to imply, the world in which I live seldom *appears* silent. Let me try to explain what I mean. In my case, silence is not absence of sound but of movement.

Suppose it is a calm day, absolutely still, not a twig or leaf stirring. To me it will seem quiet as a tomb though hedgerows are full of noisy but invisible birds. Then comes a breath of air, enough to unsettle a leaf; I will see and hear that movement like an exclamation. The illusory soundlessness has been interrupted. I see, as if I heard, a visionary noise of wind in a disturbance of foliage. Wordsworth in a late poem exactly caught the phenomenon in a remarkable line:

A soft eye-music of slow-waving boughs

which may have subconsciously derived from an equally cogent line in Coleridge's *The Eolian Harp*:

A light in sound, a sound-like power of light.

The 'sound' seen by me is not necessarily equivalent to the real one. It must often be close enough, in my case helped by a subliminal memory of things once heard. I cannot watch a gale without 'hearing' an uproar of violent movement: trees thrashing, grassblades battling and flattened; or, at sea, waves locked and staggering like all-in wrestlers – this kind of thing comes through as hubbub enough. On the other hand I also live in a world of sounds which are, as I know quite well, imaginary because non-existent. Yet for me they are part of reality. I have sometimes to make a deliberate effort to remember I am not 'hearing' anything, because there is nothing to hear. Such non-sounds include the flight and movement of birds, even fish swimming in clear water or the tank of an aquarium. I take it that the flight of most birds, at least at a distance, must be silent – bar the creaking noise made by the wings of swans and some kinds of wild geese. Yet it *appears* audible, each species creating a different 'eye-music' from the nonchalant melancholy of seagulls to the staccato flitting of tits . . .

I am now, after forty years of what we will term silence, so accommodated to it (like a hermit-crab to its shell) that were the faculty of hearing restored to me tomorrow it would appear an affliction rather than a benefit. I do not mean that I find deafness desirable but that in the course of time the disability has been assimilated to the extent that it is now an integral condition of existence, like the use of a hand. By the same token the restoration of my hearing, or the loss of my deafness, whichever is the right way of putting it, would be like having that hand cut off.

From *Deafness:A Personal Account*

Jack Ashley was an MP, with high expectations of political advancement, when at the age of forty-five he became totally deaf following a virus infection and unsuccessful surgery. Despite his deafness, he was re-elected and has become famous for his championship of the disabled.

Any person without a vital faculty like hearing is bound to feel deprived and unable to fulfil himself. My hopes and aspirations have been shattered by deafness and the course of my life radically changed. At one time my future lay in pieces with little prospect of picking them up and putting them together again. Everything, from my personal relationships with other people to my greatest ambitions were affected. Yet from this personal disaster there has emerged something which I should never have known had it not happened. The depths of human affection and kindness are not plumbed without a crisis. Nor is the veneer of superficial relationships removed so starkly under normal circumstances. Reserves, physical and mental, remain largely dormant until they are called upon to meet an urgent personal dilemma. Deafness has given me a profound appreciation of my family and real friends; an insight into the unrecognised humanity of the House of Commons; a knowledge of despair and hope I would never otherwise have known, and a greater understanding of my fellow men.

From *Journey into Silence*

My experiences are naturally different from those who were born deaf, because I have made the bleak journey from the world of hearing to the world of silence. The born deaf are denied the advantages gained by the deafened before their hearing loss, yet they are spared the desolating sense of loss. I had enjoyed the natural acquisition of speech and language and had a knowledge of the hearing world. These are priceless assets in attempting to cope with total deafness. But I was painfully and permanently aware of what I had lost. My perception of that loss is a lifelong burden.

From 'A Personal Account', in *Adjustment to Adult Hearing Loss*

*Paul West, professor and author, reflects on the challenge of
bringing up a deaf child.*

I try to keep up with the flood of periodicals, pamphlets and
reports devoted to the plight of children handicapped like, less
than, more than, you; and so I know something about flashing
clocks, volume-control handsets for telephones, BBC television
play synopses for the deaf, the Warren Wearable Walk-Away Units,
the vibrating pillow that wakes you up and the torch-like appar-
atus being designed for deaf-blind children, as well as the manual-
versus-oral teaching controversy, the Helen Keller Home in Tel-
Aviv, the Alexander Graham Bell Award given to Lyndon Baines
Johnson in 1967 'for Distinguished Service for the Deaf', the Royal
National Institute for the Deaf's bronze statuette for the Best TV
Speaker of the Year . . .

I've read about Montessori schools, the Model High School for
the Deaf, and the discoveries of Bruno Bettelheim; but the piece of
reading I most remember is an essay by a German whose special
interest is dysmelia children: deaf children without arms, and his
point was that deaf children with additional handicaps learn not
for themselves or for school, but – and this more than any other
children – for their parents. It's true of you: home is school as well
as school is, and the aim of both places is to demand the maximum
of you, to convert the world around you into your own private
hothouse. Hence, at home, all the applause you receive for saying
something such as 'thumb' and the far from rigid wooing we
subject you to. School, of course, isn't as much as home is, but you
are at home there (where you can have a birthday party and be
clapped for being 'gwd' and have a card from your teacher that says
'with luv'). School's a bit domestic, then, and home is school with a
bit more histrionic pageantry and a lewder, more ingratiating
mode of propaganda.

It's all a matter I suppose, of our being flexible enough to
encourage you into an educational opportunism, by which I mean

an opportunism, *non scholae sed vitae* (as the Latin proverb has it) – not for school but for life.

From *Words for a Deaf Daughter*

Paul West writes in a letter to the editor:

The daughter in my title is an only child, was born deaf (plus some brain damage) and attended the Royal School for the Deaf, Manchester; her intellectual progress virtually ceased with the onset of puberty, alas.

> It is hard to know how to behave with the dead; their enormous deafness and rigidity is so studied. One becomes awkward as if in the presence of royalty.
>
> Lawrence Durrell

*How Dorothy Miles came to write poetry and later to create poems
for presentation in sign language.*

These things I remember: Hills first of all – the hills of North Wales
where I was born; not the high, wild mountains of Snowdonia, but
the more domesticated hills of Flintshire, rolling down towards the
Irish Sea. The sea itself, in many different places and moods – but
chiefly the sea tamed to ebb and flow at the convenience of
holiday-makers along a stretch of 'golden sands' at the seaside
resort of Rhyl, my first remembered home. Voices – my father
singing soldiers' songs, my mother reciting narrative poems, my
eldest sister crooning lullabies at my bedside, or reading aloud the
poems she wrote herself; and the blended voices of schoolchildren,
church choirs or football crowds upraised in hymn. Music everywhere – accompanying the voices, blaring from the radio or from
the loudspeakers of the local amusement park, thumping and
per-umping from the instruments of the Rhyl Silver Prize Band, or
wafting more sedately from the orchestra pit of the Pavilion
Theatre. Theatre – song and dance and drama. The two children's
plays my mother wrote and directed, and other community plays
and pageants that various friends or members of the family were
involved in from time to time; a totally fascinating world of
make-believe and madness to which I lost my heart forever.

Then the coming of the Second World War. A brief memory of air
raid sirens being tested for a drill, and of a troop of soldiers
harmonizing in the dusk as they marched to their billets. Six
months later a sudden illness, diagnosed as cerebrospinal meningitis; and a long quiet convalescence during which I had to learn to
walk again. Afterwards, the silence that I had accepted as part of
the sick-room remained as a fact of my life.

All these sensations crowded into less than nine years; then a
different world. The deaf school in Manchester, a huge industrial
city where the air raid sirens were for real during the long nights of
the Battle of Britain. Speech lessons, interesting only if I learned a

new poem or song from them; group amplifiers that tickled my ears inside when turned up full-blast; and the sign language, Manchester version, learned from other children and enjoyed with them, but never thought of as a means of retaining communication with the receding world of my childhood.

A year after the war ended Britain established its first high school for the deaf. The Mary Hare Grammar School, far away in the South of England. A scholarship exam, passed with flying colours and I began my real education; English Literature, French, History, Algebra, Latin, and so much else, woven into four tumultuous adolescent years when I was either gloriously in love or desperately heartbroken. And by the time I left school, my family had moved to live near London, and Wales was home no longer.

Skip seven years, to Gallaudet College* in Washington, D.C., then and still the world's only liberal Arts College for a predominantly deaf student body. Thence I came in 1957, drawn by the possibility of being able to act in college productions – and there I fell in love again, this time with the American Sign Language, so much more complete and creative than the British version. It served to bring theatre and music and easy intellectual conversation firmly back into my life, and made me a whole person again. For me, there was no going back . . .

The English Language (albeit with a slight Welsh accent) was my mother-tongue. My poems are written from the words and music that still sing in my mind. Of recent years, I have tried to blend words with sign language as closely as lyrics and tunes are blended in song. In such poems, the signs I chose are a vital part of the total effect, and to understand *my* intention the poem should be seen as well as read. This is the difference between these particular poems, and those that have been written for English and are freely interpreted by individual signers.

From the 'Introduction' to *Gestures*

* Gallaudet University since 1987.

Elizabeth Quinn, the actress, was deafened by illness at the age of two. In 1981 she played the part of the deaf girl, Sarah Norman, in Children of a Lesser God *by Mark Medoff* at the Mermaid Theatre in London. The following extracts are from her autobiography written with Michael Owen.*

Reflections on Sarah Norman's opening speech

The play's action begins with Sarah's concluding lines of the argument, a despairing assessment of the state of her life which rises to a declaration of defiant independence. The speech is a curiosity in several ways as it is given in sign language only and left uninterpreted – a symbol of that defiant attitude.

American Sign Language is a free form of communication relying more on images and concepts than neat grammatical precision. It can condense a statement into a single gesture with its use of facial expression and body language. In ASL, the opening speech Elizabeth signed before making her first hasty exit from the stage would read: 'ME HAVE NOTHING. ME DEAFY. SPEECH INEPT, INTELLIGENCE – TINY BLOCKHEAD. ENGLISH – BLOW AWAY. LEFT ONE YOU. DEPEND – NO. THINK MYSELF ENOUGH. JOIN, UNJOINED . . .'

Author Medoff has offered his own translation of that speech: 'I HAVE NOTHING. NO HEARING, NO SPEECH, NO INTELLIGENCE, NO LANGUAGE. I HAVE ONLY YOU. I DON'T NEED YOU. I HAVE ME ALONE. JOIN. UNJOINED . . .'

If that speech charted the progress of Sarah Norman, Elizabeth was also aware that it was directly relevant to her own life:

It said so much about what was true to me. To be deaf and not to be able to speak. Because you have no language people always thought you were not intelligent. For so many years I did feel I had nothing. That I was less than other hearing people and could not be useful. There was an image which came to me which I used to think about in rehearsal. It was of me being

52

chained to the floor while others stood around all pointing at me. It meant I could not do anything for myself. I used to depend on so many people, too many people, and they were always men – my father, my brother Billy, lovers or directors. The last man I depended on was the director Gordon Davidson. He had helped me and led me into the play. But I knew by coming to London I was going to have to stand on my own and be independent no matter what happened. That was me – unjoined.

Again and again, the words and thoughts of Sarah Norman found an echo in her own existence. First, the anger and frustration of being passed over as a second-class citizen, denied an individuality of her own because her communication was limited. Then, on a gentler level, the innate intelligence, the almost childish sense of fun and the capacity to give love. By drawing on her own experience and bringing to it both her personal and her actress's intuition she was able to bring Sarah vibrantly to life.

From Michael Owen's Prologue

. . was intrigued by this profoundly deaf young woman, who remained steadfastly silent yet spoke with dancing hands and animated facial expression which had an eloquence of their own. I wanted to know more about the life which had brought her to such a commanding and deeply-felt performance on the stage . . .

As I have discovered through many conversations with her, Elizabeth is not just a bright and charming girl who has overcome the disadvantages which life has placed unfairly in her path. She is more complicated than that . . . If we were at odds during our discussions she would regularly remind me, 'Don't forget, English is only my second language,' American Sign Language coming definitely first . . . She is intelligent, endlessly curious and courageous, sometimes to the point of reckless folly.

That courage is reflected in her story. The world of the deaf, as I came to understand, has tensions and politics of its own which the so-called 'hearing world' too little understands. Yet even in that complex silent society, Elizabeth was an exception. She lost her hearing in early childhood but those few years were a sufficient foundation for her to be able to use her voice later, even though she could not hear it herself. She was brought up in a hearing family environment and that family, for all their several misfortunes, raised her with an attentive interest in the things of conventional life from which other deaf youngsters would be excluded.

From that family base, Elizabeth went on to spend long years in deaf institutions and social surroundings where the inhabitants had a deaf culture – held at times with defiant pride – with which she was unfamiliar and into which she remained for a long time uninvited. She was between two worlds and that factor was almost as significant as the lack of hearing itself.

Elizabeth is the product of a rare set of circumstances which have brought her often to the edge of defeat and, less frequently, to soaring elation. From years of insecurity and self-doubt she has found the confidence and self-reliance to lead a full and participating life which has allowed a concern for others to be added to the concentration on mere survival. For all the setbacks she encountered, some inner strength kept her going. Quite what the nature of that strength is lies almost beyond identification; but it has something to do with the capacity of the human spirit to prevail and to aspire, and from that we can all learn and benefit. •

From *Listen to Me – The Story of Elizabeth Quinn*

* See page 202.

*Jessica Rees was born with normal hearing, but was severely
deafened by meningitis at the age of four. She was educated at the
Mary Hare Grammar School for the Deaf. Her successful integration
with hearing students on the Outward Bound Adventure Course
described here made her decide to leave her school and continue her
education in the Sixth Form of Charterhouse School. At the age of
seventeen she was deafened totally by a hit-and-run car accident.
Nevertheless, she gained a place at Oxford.*

My life changed a few months after my mother's death, when I
went on an Outward Bound course in mid-Wales, near Towyn, for
three weeks in August 1979. Although I arrived at the Outward
Bound Centre with another deaf girl to whom I could cling for
support, we were immediately split up and put into separate
groups. The object of this was to make us come out of our shells
and speak to the other hearing students on the course instead of
just sticking to each other. It was quite true that had I been able to
talk to Gail all the time I would have virtually ignored most of the
other girls in my group on the specious grounds that I found them
difficult to lipread. As it was, I had to persevere and keep trying
while at the same time educating them to 'speak properly to me'. It
was very good for me, since I had now been at Mary Hare for four
years and was a bit too used to people looking at me all the time
while also speaking clearly. Suddenly I found myself in a group
with nine other girls who had never met a deaf person before and
none of them had any idea about how to speak to me. They either
mumbled in an embarrassed fashion or spoke far too slowly,
exaggerating their mouth movements grossly as they did so. This
only made them even more difficult to lipread since it distorted the
normal speech patterns and made the atmosphere doubly awkward
for both parties.

The first two days were awful. The rest of the group all seemed to
get to know each other much more quickly than I did. I was a
frustrated onlooker, unable to join in their conversations, unable to

55

make them understand that I wanted to converse *with* them and not to them, unable to obtain any positive feedback in any form, and unable to participate in the 'after-lights-out' chatter in the dormitory. Nobody seemed to know quite what to do with me and I didn't have the nerve to tell them. For the first time, I began to feel angry at my deafness, to such an extent that I started to have worrying visions about my future life. What if I was never able to mix with hearing people? What if I had to be segregated in a deaf ghetto for the rest of my life? I really started to think of myself as a handicapped person instead of a person in my own right who, by the way, happened to have a handicap in the form of deafness.

I did find a friend, however, in one girl in the group. She was called Claire and she had worked with various kinds of disabled people before and could see just how frustrated I was getting. She tried telling the others that I was 'quite normal really', but they still felt embarrassed and didn't quite know how they were supposed to react to my deafness. Hence by the third day I was really reaching a point where I simply couldn't continue in the same fashion for three more weeks. Something drastic was going to have to happen, and it was going to have to happen soon. I couldn't bear the tension any longer . . .

This is how I managed to do it, and in fact it was far easier than I thought it would be. On the evening of the third day I was miserably making the tea for our group in the kitchen and I involuntarily caught sight of my reflection in the mirror. I was fairly disgusted with the girl I saw, so I gave her a long talking to:

'You're a fine one aren't you? Just because you're deaf, you sit there blaming everybody else under the sun for it. As if it mattered! You think that just because you're a little bit weak in the ears your whole life is automatically wasted and that's it. Well, I'm telling you, young lady, *you* should know all about wasting your life – you're really going the right way for that. And it isn't your handicap or your mother's death that's causing it. You're doing this to yourself.'

After that, I decided I was going to take a really long, hard look at myself. A handicap is as big as you allow it to be and I decided that I was not going to let my deafness stop me from having a good three weeks on this course.

It was a very simply executed plan. I just picked up a chair from the kitchen and walked out to where the rest of the group were sitting. I then plunged right into the centre of their social circle, put down the chair and sat on it hard. I told them, 'Now listen, you lot. You can't ignore me just because I'm deaf any longer,' and I waited.

They were amazed. Some people looked away or at each other with embarrassed smiles. One girl got up muttering something about a 'phone call. I belted at her at the top of my voice, 'SIT DOWN!' Then I continued.

'I want to talk with you and join in instead of being the passive parasite I feel at present. So I'm going to talk and if you don't answer I shall GET VERY VERY ANGRY.' One girl told me I was being difficult and that being deaf I shouldn't have come on the Outward Bound course. She was instantly rebuked by Claire who told her *she* was being difficult and also extremely narrow-minded. One by one the rest of the group joined in and told her to give me a chance. She was suitably chastened and mumbled an apology. Furthermore the rest of the group, having stuck up for me, seemed less uncomfortable than before. We now had a common alliance. 'Why don't you ask me questions?' I proposed, 'and if you stop I will start asking you questions but some of them might be very embarrassing.' The last two words were said in a more threatening tone than the rest.

There was no need for me to do anything else after that. They bombarded me with questions and I was not given a break. Later Claire told me that they had been so surprised at just what I had done to make them notice me, they couldn't bear to think what sort of intimate questions I might ask them straight out in front of everyone else, given half a chance.

After this I got on really well with the other girls in the group and they all became much more understanding about my deafness. If an order was issued (or even more important a warning) they made sure that I heard it. The problem was that often neither member of the group would trust another to tell me so I ended up getting the same order relayed to me nine times in a row.

From *Sing a Song of Silence*

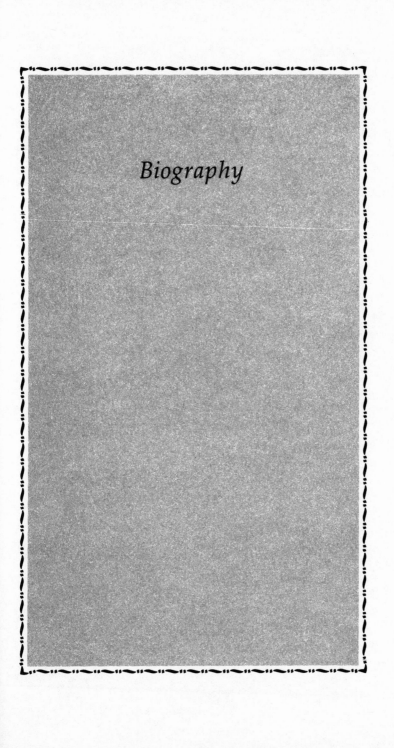

Biography

Henry Gurney, first head of a well-known Norfolk Quaker family, was troubled by deafness in middle-age and wrote about some contemporary 'remedies'.

Ellen [his wife] held the purse strings and, as Henry ruefully observed:

> When as he doth for any money ask
> for needful use as either debts to pay
> Our subsidy, town charges, or the tasks
> which may not bid denial or delay
> Although she doth not flatly them deny
> Yet pays them not without some cross reply.*

On top of this Henry found that he was going really deaf. This may have been a convenience at home, but it made his attendance at Court almost useless . . .

He mentions a remedy for deafness tried by the miller of Great Ellingham who had been deaf for three months through 'an noyse in his head which letted him to hear his mill clapper being in the mill'. In the month of May before the sun rose the miller took the dew from the grass by skimming it with his hand and pouring it into his ear, working it in with his little finger. This he did for a month. Then, 'in a sudden rush or flash, the wind breezed out of his head and he was cured'. Henry writes, 'Myself never tried this because my deafness is not by a wynde.'

Another remedy was sent to him by Lord North, 'who was taken stone deaf so as he could not hear by no means any speech' but was healed by obeying these instructions: 'Bake a little loaf of bean flour and while hot rive it into halves and into each half pour into three or four spoonsful of bitter almonds – then clap both the halves to both the ears on going to bed and keep them close and keep your head warm.'

Perhaps Henry was healed, too, for his spirits took a turn for the better when the Norfolk coast was fortified against the Spanish

Armada, whose defeat he describes with great verve soon after the event.

From *Friends and Relation*

* This and subsequent quotations are from 'The Commonplace Book o Register of Henry Gurney', manuscript in the Bodleian Library Oxford.

> I found that of the senses, the eye is the most superficial, the ear the most arrogant, smell the most voluptuous, taste the most superstitious and fickle, touch the most profound and philosophical.†
>
> Denis Diderot

† Translated by Helen Keller and quoted with approval in her essay 'Value of the Senses'.

A meeting between Edward Bone and one Kempe, both 'defected'
with deafness, a long time ago.

EDWARD BONE, of Ladcock in this county, was servant to Mr Courtney therein. He was deaf from his cradle, and consequently dumb (Nature cannot give out where it hath not received) yet could learn, and express to his master, any news that was stirring in the country. Especially, if there went speech of a sermon within some miles' distance, he would repair to the place with the soonest, and setting himself directly against the preacher, look him steadfastly in the face while his sermon lasted; to which religious zeal his honest life was also answerable. Assisted with a firm memory, he would not only know any party whom he had once seen for ever after, but also make him known to any other, by some special observation and difference. There was one Kempe, not living far off, defected accordingly, on whose meetings there were such embracements, such strange, often and earnest tokenings, and such hearty laughters and other passionate gestures, that their want of a tongue seemed rather an hindrance to others conceiving them, than to their conceiving one another.

From Fuller's *The Worthies of England*

William Holder, the first English educator of the deaf, was an erudite
cleric. He was elected a Fellow of the Royal Society and wrote
Elements of Deaf Speech *as well as various treatises on harmony*
and the Julian calendar.

He is a handsome, gracefull person, and of a delicate constitution, and of an even and smooth temper; so that, if one would goe about to describe a perfect good man, would drawe this Doctor's Character. He is very Musicall, both theoretically and practically, and he had a sweet voyce: gracefull Elocution; his discourse so Gent. and obligeing; cleer reason; is a good Poet. He is extremely well qualified for his place of the Sub-Almoner of the King's Chapell, being a person abhorring covetousness, and full of Pitty.

The only Son of Edward Popham, Admirall for the Parliament, being borne deafe and dumbe, was sent to him to learne to speake, which he taught him to doe: by what method, and how soon, you may see in the Appendix concerning it to his *Elements of Speech*. It is a most ingeniose and curious Discourse, and untouched by any other; he was beholding to no Author; did only consult with Nature. This Gentleman's son afterwards was a little while (upon Dr Holder's preferment to Ely) a scholar of Dr Wallis* (a most ill-natured man, an egregious lyer and backbiter, a flatterer and fawner . . .) under whom he forgott what he learnt before, the child not enduring his morose pedantique humour . . .

Mr Thomas Hobbes writes to me, I wonder not if Dr Wallis, or any other, that have studyed Mathematicks onely to gaine Preferment, when his ignorance is discovered, convert his study to jugling and to the gaining of a reputation of conjuring, decyphering, and such Arts. As for the matter it selfe, I meane the teaching of a man borne deafe and dumbe to speake, I thinke it impossible. But I doe not count him deafe and indocible [unteachable] that can heare a word spoken as loud as is possible at the very entrance to his Eare; and he that could make him heare (being a great and common good) would well deserve both to be honoured and to be

enriched. He that could make him speake a few words onely
deserved nothing. But he that brags of this and cannot doe it,
deserves to be whipt.

But to returne to this honest worthy Gentleman – Anno about
1646, he went to Bletchington to his parsonage, where his hospital-
ity and learning, mixt with great courtesie, easily conciliated the
love of all his neighbours to him.

From Aubrey's *Brief Lives*

* See pages 83-84.

My wings are folded o'er mine ears,
My wings are crossed o'er mine eyes,
Yet through their silver shade appears,
And through their lulling plumes arise,
A shape, a throng of sounds.*

Percy Bysshe Shelley

* These lines from *Prometheus Unbound* are Helen Keller's introductory
quotation to her *Chant of Darkness*.

Bulwer-Lytton combined literary fame as author of a variety of works with distinction in politics. He was appointed a minister by Disraeli in 1858.

Lytton possessed a marvellously strong will, and had a faith in himself which almost amounted to genius. He seems to have made up his mind that he would compel the world to confess him capable of playing the part of a politician. He was deaf, and his articulation was so defective that most people who heard him speak in public for the first time found themselves unable to understand him. Such difficulties would assuredly have scared any ordinary man out of the Parliamentary arena for ever. But Lytton seems to have determined that he would make a figure in Parliament. He set himself to public speaking as coolly as if he were a man, like Gladstone or Bright, whom nature had marked out for such a competition by her physical gifts. He became a decided, and even in a certain sense, a great success. He could not strike into a debate actually going on; his defects of hearing shut him off from such a performance; and no man who is not a debater will ever hold a really high position in the House of Commons. But he could review a previous night's arguments in a speech abounding in splendid phrases and brilliant illustrations. He could pass for an orator. He actually did so . . .

From *A Short History of our Own Times*

Lester Piggott's* parents discover that their son is deaf.

'I think,' said the ear-nose-and-throat man, 'that your son is deaf.'

The parents were astounded and disbelieving. 'He can't be,' they said. 'He hears what we say. He answers us.'

'He hears a little,' they were told, 'but he is very bright, and he lip-reads.'

Iris and Keith still didn't believe him.

'I'll show you,' the doctor said. He got Lester to stand at his knees, and asked him a simple question. Lester answered without hesitation.

'He's not deaf,' Keith asserted.

The doctor shook his head, picked up a large sheet of paper and held it in front of his mouth so that Lester could see only his eyes looking over the top. He asked Lester another question, just as simple. Lester gave no sign at all of having heard. The doctor put down the paper and asked the same question again. Lester answered at once.

This demonstration, once or twice repeated with exactly the same results, reluctantly convinced the Piggotts ...

The difficulty with hearing and the fact of his being an only child combined powerfully from the start to turn him inwards to himself. Add to this natural isolation a focus of interest, and you have all the ingredients of super-single-mindedness. He saw horses all around him: they were his father's job, his mother's interest, his family's tradition. The barrier of deafness kept most of the world away as if in the misty distance.

From *Lester*

* England's famous Champion Jockey.

Letters and Essays

Beethoven realised in his late twenties that he was becoming deaf. At the time he was primarily a virtuoso pianist; a career which he had to abandon as his deafness got worse. Most of his music was written when his hearing was seriously impaired. During his last ten years, when he was totally deaf, he composed many of his greatest works, including the Ninth Symphony, the Missa Solemnis *and his last four string quartets. The document which follows, written in a mood of despair, was found among the composer's papers after his death and is known as the 'Heiligenstadt Testament'.*

Heiligenstadt, 6 October 1802

O my fellow men, who consider me, or describe me as unfriendly, peevish or even misanthropic, how greatly do you wrong me. For you do not know the secret reason why I appear to you to be so. Ever since my childhood my heart and soul have been imbued with the tender feeling of goodwill; and I have always been ready to perform even great actions. But just think, for the last six years I have been afflicted with an incurable complaint which has been made worse by incompetent doctors. From year to year my hopes of being cured have gradually been shattered and finally I have been forced to accept the prospect of a *permanent infirmity* (the curing of which may perhaps take years or may even prove to be impossible). Though endowed with a passionate and lively temperament and even fond of the distractions offered by society I was soon obliged to seclude myself and live in solitude. If at times I decided just to ignore my infirmity, alas! how cruelly was I then driven back by the intensified sad experience of my poor hearing. Yet I could not bring myself to say to people: 'Speak up, shout, for I am deaf.' Alas! how could I possibly refer to the impairing *of a sense* which in me should be more perfectly developed than in other people, a sense which at one time I possessed in the greatest perfection, even to a degree of perfection such as assuredly few in my profession possess or have ever possessed – Oh, I cannot do it; so forgive me, if you ever see me withdrawing from your company which I used to enjoy. Moreover my misfortune pains me doubly, inasmuch as it leads to my being misjudged. For me there can be no relaxation in human society, no refined conversations, no mutual confidences. I must live quite alone and may creep into society only as often as sheer necessity demands; I must live like an outcast. If I appear in company I am overcome by a burning anxiety, a fear that I am running the risk of letting people notice my condition – And that has been my experience during the last six months which I have spent in the country. My sensible doctor by suggesting that I should spare my hearing as much as possible has more or less encouraged my present natural inclination, though indeed when carried away now and then by my instinctive desire for human society, I have let myself be tempted to seek it. But how humiliated I have felt if somebody standing beside me heard the sound of a flute in the distance and *I heard nothing*, or if somebody heard *a shepherd sing* and again I heard nothing – Such experiences almost made me despair, and I was on the point of putting an end to my life – The only thing that held me back was *my art*. For indeed it seemed to me impossible to leave this world before I had produced all the works that I felt the urge to compose; and thus I have dragged on this miserable existence – a truly miserable existence, seeing that I have such a sensitive body that any fairly sudden change can plunge me from the best spirits into the worst of humours – *Patience*, that is the virtue, I am told, which I must now choose for my guide; and I now possess it – I hope that I shall persist in my resolve to endure to the end, until it pleases the inexorable Parcae [Fates] to cut the thread; perhaps my condition will improve, perhaps not; at any rate I am now resigned – At the early age of 28 I was obliged to become a philosopher, though this was not easy; for indeed this is more difficult for an artist than for anyone else – Almighty God, who look down into my innermost soul, you see into my heart and you know that it is filled with love for humanity and a desire to do good. Oh my fellow men, when some day you read this statement, remember that you have done me wrong; and let some unfortunate man derive comfort from the thought that he has found another equally unfortunate who, notwithstanding all the obstacles imposed by nature, yet did everything in his power to be raised to the rank of noble artists and human beings. – And you, my brothers Carl and [Johann], when I am dead, request on my behalf Professor Schmidt, if he is still living, to describe my disease, and attach this written document to his record, so that after my death at any rate the world and I may be reconciled as far as possible – At the same time I herewith nominate you both heirs to my small property (if I may so describe it) – Divide it honestly, live in harmony and help one another . . . Farewell and love one another . . . – Well, that is all – joyfully I go to meet Death – should it come before I have had an opportunity of developing all my artistic gifts, then in spite of my hard fate it would still come too soon, and no doubt I would like it to postpone its coming – Yet even so I should be content, for would it not free me from a condition of continual suffering? Come then, Death, *whenever* you like, and with courage I will go to meet you – Farewell; and when I am dead, do not wholly forget me. I deserve to be remembered by you, since during my lifetime I have often thought of you and tried to make you happy – Be happy –

Ludwig van Beethoven

Heiligenstadt, 10 October 1802 – Thus I take leave of you – and, what is more, rather sadly – yes, the hope I cherished – the hope I brought with me here of being cured to a certain extent at any rate – that hope I must now abandon completely. As the autumn leaves fall and wither, likewise – that hope has faded for me. I am leaving here – almost in the same condition as I arrived – Even that high courage – which has often inspired me on fine summer days – has vanished – Oh Providence – do but grant me one day *of pure joy* – For so long now the inner echo of real joy has been unknown to me – Oh when – oh when, Almighty God – shall I be able to hear and feel this echo again in the temple of Nature and in contact with humanity – Never? – No! – Oh, that would be too hard.

From *The Letters of Beethoven*, translated by Emily Anderson.

Castle Square, Tuesday, 27 December 1808

We spent Friday evening with our friends at the boardinghouse, and our curiosity was gratified by the sight of their fellow-inmates, Mrs Drew and Miss Hook, Mr Wynne and Mr Fitzhugh; the latter is brother to Mrs Lance, and very much the gentleman. He has lived in that house more than twenty years, and, poor man! is so totally deaf that they say he could not hear a cannon were it fired close to him; having no cannon at hand to make the experiment, I took it for granted, and talked to him a little with my fingers, which was funny enough. I recommended him to read Corinna.*

From a letter to her sister Cassandra

* A novel by Mme de Staël published in 1807.

26 November 1882

On Friday morning . . . I arrived about 7 or 8 o'clock from Paris, after five days' stay – five of the most remarkable days of my life. On Monday (as you may have seen in *The Times*) I was invited to dinner at Victor Hugo's, and accordingly presented myself in a state of perturbation as well as delight before the greatest – I know – and I believe the best, man now living. No words can express his kindness of manner, as he said on taking my hand, 'Je suis heureux de vous serrer la main comme à mon fils.' I am delighted to say that he is even more wonderful – all things considered – for his age than Mrs Proctor for hers. He will be eighty-one in February, and walked upright and firm without a stick. His white hair is as thick as his dark eyebrows, and his eyes are as bright and clear as a little child's. After dinner, he drank my health with a little speech, of which – tho' I sat just opposite him – my accursed deafness prevented my hearing a single word. This, however, was the only drawback – tho' certainly a considerable one – to my pleasure.* On Wednesday evening I went . . . to the Théâtre Français . . . the second night of the representation, on a Parisian stage, of a play which had first been acted on the same day fifty years before, and suppressed on the next day by Louis Philippe's government, on account of a supposed allusion, in a single line, to the infamy of Citizen Philippe Egalité, that worthy monarch's worthy parent . . . it was generally very fine, as far as a deaf wretch can judge.

From a letter to his mother

* In his biography of *Swinburne* (1974) Philip Henderson gives the following account of the toasts after dinner: 'Unfortunately, Swinburne was unable to hear the terms in which the great poet proposed his health and Hugo was equally deaf to Swinburne's fervent reply. Swinburne then drained his glass to the Master and dashed it to the ground. But we are told that Hugo, misunderstanding this traditional gesture, only mourned the loss of one of his best wine glasses.'

75

Stanhope Gardens, 21 April 1950

Last night I was thinking 'If I could jump out of the window one bang and I'd be out of it.' For this is the sixth floor.

Then I thought of Max's story of the old lady who went to church with her ear trumpet. And so the stern Scotch sexton or verger or something, eyed her a bit. Then he said 'Madam one toot and you're oot.' Perhaps that's what it would be like, One toot and you're oot.

From a letter to Peggy Kirkaldy

HE THAT HATH EARS, LET HIM TALK

It is a moot point whether people suffer worst, if the disadvantages they struggle under are obvious to all, like weighing 24 stone or having an albatross around the neck; or if they are invisible, like gallstones or a guilty conscience. But certainly the invisible ailments are the more likely to be misunderstood by others; and one of the most misunderstood is deafness.

Bandage your eyes for a day, and the drawbacks are immediate: you cannot read or write and you bump into things. Put plugs in your ears, however, and all you may feel to begin with is a welcome absence of the noise of other people's sports cars. Yet in the long run deafness is just as bad as blindness, because it cuts one off from *people*.

A blind person does not make *us* uncomfortable. We may help him across a road, but otherwise he demands no more of the rest of us than he would if he could see. But deafness incommodes us with the effort to make ourselves understood – so most of us simply make three minutes' polite conversation and then talk to someone else. Add that up over a lifetime and it makes a pit of loneliness.

The National Health Service would be justified, to my mind, if only by the number of people who heard voices for the first time in 25 years with a free hearing aid; but there are plenty of forms of deafness to which even the best machine can give only, in the old phrase, all aid short of help.

Sign language is no use unless the other person knows the signs – which means, in practice, only other deaf people or those who have spent long hours ignoring the sermon in school chapel. Even lip-reading has snags. It is hard to follow a general conversation – whatever the spy stories say, no one can read a bearded stranger across a darkened café. And much of it remains guesswork: 'The beer pail is a-fillin' being literally indistinguishable from 'The mere male is a villain' – so it works only if the deaf person is fairly bright.

Whatever the method, talking to the deaf does take some imagination – if only to realise that they do not all need the same thing. Some, for example, hear voices better across other noises (unlikely as that seems): when my mother was going deaf there was a stage when she was at her best in the Tube, and some of the most ardent crises of our adolescence had to be discussed at the tops of our voices going round and round and round the Inner Circle. If someone has a hearing aid, there is more point in clarity than in bellowing – which simply makes you sound like those station voices announcing that the boo-fifteen will leave from platform blah.

What you say can be as important as how you speak it: it helps if you begin with the subject you are going to talk about, and if you get stuck repeat the whole phrase, and not just one word – monosyllables are hard to take in, and rephrasing a thing in childish language only makes things worse – it's their hearing that is dicey, not their understanding.

Even people with aids need to see the speaker, and lip-readers need a good light and steady speech – which might seem too obvious to mention, except that it is always my mother's most intelligent friends who seem least capable of slowing down, facing front and taking the fag out of their mouths when they speak to her. And the deaf person must know a conversation is going to start, so that he can turn on the aid, put on his glasses, stop filling a hot-water bottle or whatever – I remember a conversation between one man and his deaf wife: 'We were quarrelling . . .' 'Oh James, we weren't *quarrelling!*' 'Well, *I* was, but you wouldn't look!'

Too often, indeed, the deaf do give the impression that they are refusing to look, rejecting contact – but this is just the defensive shell of anyone who has been snubbed too often. My mother, who is an ace lip-reader, says people are incredibly kind if you say straight out – 'I'm deaf. Please speak slowly.'

'The trouble is that it doesn't show,' one of them said. 'It would almost be easier if your ears turned purple or something.' At least purple ears would stop the commonest affront the deaf have to take: that people, misunderstanding their deafness, think they are stupid. We do the same to foreigners if we are not careful: and most people know the gloom of being in a country where we hardly know the language – for a few minutes people speak to us like children and then the talk rockets on and leaves us out altogether. In this, the deaf are strangers in their own country for ever.

The troubles of the deaf are not, primarily, to be solved by money and good works. Of course it is nice when a hard-of-hearing group gets a minibus to tootle it around the countryside and deaf children's schools need money for equipment and teachers. But even the National Deaf Children's Society reckons that the attitude of hearing people is the core of the problem. If people included them in, deafness would be a bearable disability. As it is, it is one of the worst. So send no money, knit no blankets, get up no church bazaars. Just *talk* to them. That'll do it.

From the *Observer*, 21 November 1971

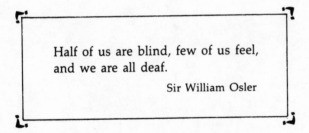

Half of us are blind, few of us feel, and we are all deaf.

Sir William Osler

Fiction

*Duncan Campbell, the principal character of this documentary
novel, was a real person, equally famous for his 'second sense' as for
his conquest of deafness which some contemporaries believed
to be feigned.*

If any learned man should have advanced this proposition, that
mere human art could give to the deaf man what should be equal to
his hearing, and to the dumb man an equivalent for his want of
speech, so that he should converse as freely almost as other hearing
or talking persons; that he might, though born deaf, be by art
taught how to read, write, and understand any language, as well as
students that have their hearing, would not the world, and many
even of the learned part of it, say that nothing could be more
extravagantly wild, more mad and frantic? The learned Dr Wallis,*
geometry professor of Oxford, did first of all lay down this
proposition, and was counted by many to have overshot the point
of learning, and to have been the author of a whimsical thesis . . .
. . . should I come afterwards and say, that there is now living a
deaf and dumb man, and born so, who could by his own genius
teach all others deaf and dumb to read, write and converse with the
talking and hearing part of mankind, some would, I warrant, very
religiously conclude, that I was about to introduce some strange
new miracle-monger and imposter into the world, with a design of
setting up some new sect of anti-Christianism, as formidable as
that of Brachmans. Should I proceed still farther and say, that this
same person, so deaf and dumb, might be able also to show a
presaging power, or kind of prophetical genius (if I may be allowed
the expression) by telling any strange persons he never saw before
in his life, their names at first sight in writing, and by telling them
the past actions of their lives, and predicting to them determined
truths of future contengencies, . . . would not they conclude that I
was going to usher in a new Mahomet?
Since therefore, there does exist such a man in London, who
actually is deaf and dumb, and was born so; who does write and

read, and converse with anybody; who likewise can, by a presaging gift, set down in writing the name of any stranger at first sight, tell him his past actions, and predict his future occurences in fortune; and since he has practised this talent as a profession with great success for a long series of years upon innumerable persons in every state and vocation in life, from the peeress to the waiting-woman, and from the lady mayoress to the milliner and sempstress, will it not be wonderfully entertaining to give the world a perfect history of this so singular a man's life?

From the Introduction to
*History of the Life and Adventures
of Mr Duncan Campbell*

* Dr Wallis, who was Defoe's brother-in-law and died in 1703, was one of the first English teachers of the deaf. He claimed to have been the first, but most of his contemporaries did not accept his claim, doubted his skill, and preferred William Holder'st credentials. Defoe's novel which goes into great detail about Dr Wallis's methods, is of historical interest as it is the first novel bringing to the notice of the general public the possibility of educating the profoundly deaf.

† See page 64.

Fenella, 'deaf and dumb' train-bearer to the Countess of Derby, is secretly in love with Julian Peveril. King Charles by a cunning ruse exposes her as a fraud and spy.

Will your ladyship forgive me?' said Charles. 'I have studied your sex long – I am mistaken if your little maiden is not as capable of caring for herself as any of us.'

'Impossible!' said the Countess.

'Possible, and most true,' whispered the King. 'I will instantly convince you of the fact, though the experiment is too delicate to be made by any but your ladyship. Yonder she stands, looking as if she heard no more than the marble pillar against which she leans. Now, if Lady Derby will contrive either to place her hand near the region of the damsel's heart, or at least on her arm, so that she can feel the sensation of the blood when the pulse increases, then do you, my Lord Ormond, beckon Julian Peveril out of sight – I will show you in a moment that it can stir at sounds spoken.'

The Countess, much surprised, afraid of some embarrassing pleasantry on the part of Charles, yet unable to repress her curiosity, placed herself near Fenella, as she called her little mute; and, while making signs to her, contrived to place her hand on her wrist.

At this moment the King, passing near them, said 'This is a horrid deed – the villain Christian has stabbed young Peveril!'

The mute evidence of the pulse, which bounded as if a cannon had been discharged close to the poor girl's ear, was accompanied by such a loud scream of agony, as distressed, while it startled, the good-natured monarch himself. 'I did but jest,' he said; 'Julian is well, my pretty maiden. I only used the wand of a certain blind deity, called Cupid, to bring a deaf and dumb vassal of his to the exercise of her faculties.'

'I am betrayed!' she said, with her eyes fixed on the ground – 'I am betrayed! and it is fit that she whose life has been spent in practising treason on others, should be caught in her own snare.'*

From *Peveril of the Peak*

85

* Scott used this situation again in *The Talisman* and it is also found in Boccaccio's *Decameron* (First Tale, Third Day) and in Tobias Smollett's *Peregrine Pickle*.

The most happy marriage I can picture or imagine to myself would be the union of a deaf man to a blind woman.†

Attributed to Samuel Taylor Coleridge by Thomas Allsop‡

† The same thought occurs elsewhere: 'There neuer shal be chiding in that house, where the man is blynd and the woman deafe' (from *Florio His First Fruites*, 1578); 'Then marriage may be said to be past in all quietness, when the wife is blynd and the husband deafe' (from John Heywood's *Collection of English Proverbs*).

‡ The third edition of Thomas Allsop's *Letters, Conversations and Recollections of S.T. Coleridge* (1864) has this footnote: 'Whilst these pages are passing through the press, this most extraordinary conjunction has taken place at Barming near Maidstone.'

*Emma Woodhouse, during a social call on Mrs and Miss Bates
praises the handwriting of Jane Fairfax, Miss Bates's niece, from
whom a letter had arrived that morning. Miss Bates is the
kindly garrulous daughter of Mrs Bates, the widow of the late
vicar of Highbury.*

You are extremely kind,' replied Miss Bates highly gratified; 'You
re such a judge, and write so beautifully yourself. I am sure there
s nobody's praise that could give us so much pleasure as Miss
Woodhouse's. My mother does not hear; she is a little deaf you
now. Ma'am,' addressing her, 'do you hear what Miss Woodhouse
s so obliging to say about Jane's handwriting?'

And Emma had the advantage of hearing her own silly com-
liment repeated twice over before the good old lady could
omprehend it. She was pondering, in the meanwhile, upon the
ossibility, without seeming very rude, of making her escape from
ane Fairfax's letter, and had almost resolved on hurrying away
irectly under some slight excuse, when Miss Bates turned to her
gain and seized her attention.

'My mother's deafness is very trifling you see – just nothing at
ll. By only raising my voice, and saying anything two or three
imes over, she is sure to hear; but then she is used to my voice. But
t is very remarkable that she should always hear Jane better than
he does me. Jane speaks so distinct! However, she will not find
er grandmamma at all deafer, than she was two years ago; which
s saying a great deal at my mother's time of life –' . . .

*Miss Bates, accompanied by Jane Fairfax, visits Mr Woodhouse and
his daughter Emma to announce the news of the engagement of Mr
Elton, the incumbent vicar, to a Miss Hawkins of Bath.*

A new neighbour for us all, Miss Woodhouse!' said Miss Bates
oyfully; 'my mother is so pleased! – she says she cannot bear to
ave the poor old Vicarage without a mistress. This is great news,

indeed. Jane, you have never seen Mr Elton! – no wonder that yo have such a curiosity to see him.'

Jane's curiosity did not appear of that absorbing nature as wholl to occupy her.

'No – I have never seen Mr Elton,' she replied, starting on thi appeal; 'is he – is he a tall man?'

'Who shall answer that question?' cried Emma. 'My father woul say "yes", Mr Knightly, "no"; and Miss Bates and I that he is jus the happy medium. When you have been here a little longer, Mis Fairfax, you will understand that Mr Elton is the standard o perfection in Highbury, both in person and mind.'

'Very true, Miss Woodhouse, so she will. He is the very bes young man – But, my dear Jane, if you remember, I told yo yesterday he was precisely the height of Mr Perry. Miss Hawkins, I dare say, an excellent young woman. His extreme attention to m mother – wanting her to sit in the vicarage-pew, that she migh hear the better, for my mother is a little deaf, you know – it is no much, but she does not hear quite quick. Jane says that Colone Campbell is a little deaf. He fancied bathing might be good for it the warm bath – but she says it did him no lasting benefit. Colone Campbell, you know, is quite our angel.'

From *Emm*

Zig-zag justice at the Old Bailey.

'Evidence, Mr Gurney!' said the sheriff, 'how little you know of the Old Bailey! – why if these London juries were to wait to consider evidence, we should never get through the business – the way we do here, is to make a zig-zag of it.'

I did not exactly comprehend the term as it was now applied . . . and I therefore made no scruple of expressing my ignorance.

'Don't you understand, Sir?' said the sheriff – 'why the next prisoner will be found guilty – the last was acquitted – the one after the next will be acquitted too – it comes alternate like – save half – convict half – that's what we call a zig-zag; and taking the haggregate, it comes to the same pint, and I think justice is done as fair here as in any court in Christendom.'

This explanation rendered the next prisoner who made his appearance, an object of considerable interest to me. He was a little dirty boy, who stood charged with having stolen a pound of bacon and a peg-top from a boy somewhat his junior. The young prosecutor produced a witness, who, as far as appearances went, might without any great injustice have taken the place of the prisoner, and who gave his evidence with considerable fluency and flippancy. His manner attracted the notice of one of the leading barristers of the Court, Mr Flappertrap, who in cross-examining him, inquired whether he knew the nature of the oath.

'Yes, I does,' said the boy.

'Explain it,' said Flappertrap.

'You may be d——d,' replied the lad, 'that's a hoath, arn't it?'

'What does he say?' said the Judge – who, as I about this period discovered, was as deaf as a post.

'He says, "you may be d——d," my Lord,' said Flappertrap, who appeared particularly glad of an opportunity to borrow a phrase, which he might use for the occasion.

'What does he mean by that?' said the Judge.

'That is the way, my Lord, in which he exhibits his knowledge of the nature of an oath.'

89

'Pah! Pah!' said the Judge – 'Boy, d'ye hear me?'

'Yes,' said the boy, 'I hears.'

'Have you ever been to school?'

'Yes,' said the boy, 'in St. Giles's parish for three years.'

'Do you know your catechism?'

The boy muttered something which was not audible to the Court generally, and was utterly lost upon the Judge personally.

'What does he say?' said his Lordship.

'Speak up, Sir,' said Mr Flappertrap.

The boy muttered again, looking down and seeming embarrassed.

'Speak louder, Sir,' said another barrister, whose name I did not know, but who was remarkable for a most unequivocal obliquity of vision – 'speak to his Lordship – look at him – look as *I* do, Sir.'

'I can't,' said the boy, 'you squints!'

A laugh followed this bit of *naiveté*, which greatly abashed the counsellor and somewhat puzzled the Judge.

'What does he say?' said his Lordship.

'He says he knows his catechism, my Lord.'

'Oh – does not know his catechism – why then what — '

'*Does* know, my Lord,' whispered the Lord Mayor, who was in the chair.

'Oh – ah – *does* know – I know – here, boy,' said his Lordship, 'you know your catechism, do you?'

'Yes,' replied he sullenly.

'We'll see, then – what is your name?' said his Lordship.

'My name,' said the intelligent lad – 'what, in the catechism?'

'Yes, what is your name?'

'M or N as the case may be,' said the boy.

'Go down, go down,' said the Judge angrily, and down he went.

'Gentlemen of the jury,' said his Lordship, 'this case will require very little of your attention – the only evidence against the prisoner at the bar which goes to fasten the crime upon him, is that which has been offered by the last witness, who evidently is ignorant of the nature and obligation of an oath. With respect to the pig's toes which the prisoner stands charged with stealing — '

'A peg-top, my Lord!' said Flappertrap, standing up, turning round, and speaking over the bench into the Judge's ears.

'Peg-top,' said his Lordship – 'oh – ah – I see – very bad pen – it looks in my notes like pig's toes. Well – peg-top – of the peg-top which it is alleged he took from the prosecutor, there has not been one syllable mentioned by the prosecutor himself; nor do I see that the charge of taking the bacon is by any means proved. There is no point for me to direct your attention to, and you will say whether the prisoner at the bar is guilty or not; and a very trumpery case it is altogether, that I must admit.'

His Lordship ceased, and the Jury again laid their heads together; again the foreman gave the little 'hem' of conscious readiness for decision; again did the clerk of the arraigns ask the important question, 'How say ye, gentlemen, is the prisoner at the bar guilty or not guilty?' 'Guilty,' said the foreman to the clerk of the arraigns; and 'I told you so,' said the sheriff to me.

From *Gilbert Gurney*

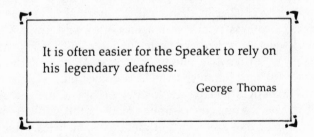

It is often easier for the Speaker to rely on his legendary deafness.

George Thomas

91

Quasimodo the deaf and hunchbacked bellringer of Notre-Dame is charged with criminal offences in the Magistrates' Court of Paris, presided over by Maître Florian, a deaf magistrate known by the title of 'auditor'. The year is 1482.

... Maître Florian, the auditor, was leafing intently through the documents of the charge laid against Quasimodo, which the clerk had held out to him, and, having glanced at them, he seemed to reflect for a moment. Thanks to this precaution, which he was always careful to take when proceeding to an interrogation, he knew in advance the names, titles and crimes of the accused, could make predictable rejoinders to predictable answers, and could survive all the ins and outs of the interrogation without letting his deafness show overmuch. For him the documents of the case were like the blind man's guide-dog. If it happened now and again that his infirmity was revealed by an incoherent apostrophe or an unintelligible question, then some ascribed this to his profundity, others to his imbecility. In either case, the honour of the magistrature was preserved, since it is better for a judge to be thought profound or an imbecile than deaf. So he took great pains to conceal his deafness from the general notice, and normally succeeded so well that he had even come to deceive himself. Which is, as it happens, easier than one might think. All hunchbacks hold their heads high, all stammerers make speeches, all deaf people talk quietly. He thought merely that his hearing was somewhat rebellious. That was the one concession he made in the matter to public opinion, during those moments of candour when he examined his conscience.

Having thus ruminated on Quasimodo's case, he threw back his head and half closed his eyes, so as to look more impartial and majestic, with the result that at that moment he was both deaf and blind. Twin conditions without which there can be no perfect judge. In this magisterial pose, he began the interrogation.

'Your name?'

But here was a circumstance which had not been 'foreseen by the law', whereby one deaf man would have to question another.

Quasimodo, totally ignorant that a question had been addressed to him, continued to stare fixedly at the judge and did not answer. The judge, who was deaf and totally ignorant of the deafness of the defendant, thought he had replied, as defendants generally did, and continued, with his stupid and mechanical self-assurance:

'Good. Your age?'

Quasimodo did not reply to this question either. The judge thought it had been answered and went on.

'Now, your trade?'

Still the same silence. The audience, meanwhile, had begun to whisper and exchange glances.

'That will do,' went on the imperturbable auditor, assuming that the defendant had completed his third reply. 'You are accused before us: *primo*, of nocturnal disturbance; *secundo*, of an unlawful act of violence against the person of a loose woman, *in praejudicium meretricis* [to the detriment of a harlot]; *tertio*, of insubordination and disloyalty towards the archers of the ordinance of the king our master. Justify yourself on all these points. Clerk, have you written down what the defendant has said so far?'

At this luckless question, a roar of laughter went up from clerks and spectators alike, so violent, so wild, so contagious, and so universal that the two deaf men could not but be aware of it. Quasimodo turned round with a scornful shrug of his hump-back, while Maître Florian, equally amazed and supposing the laughter to have been provoked by some irreverent rejoinder from the prisoner, made visible for him by that shrug of the shoulders, apostrophized him indignantly.

'The answer you have just given, you scoundrel, deserves the noose. Do you know to whom you are speaking?'

Which outburst was not calculated to stay the general explosion of merriment. Everyone found it so incongruous and absurd that the uncontrollable laughter spread even to the serjeants from the Parloir-aux-Bourgeois, those knaves of spades, as it were, whose stupidity was part of their uniform. Quasimodo alone remained unsmiling for the good reason that he understood nothing of what was going on around him . . .

. . . the clerk, just as Maître Florian Barcedienne was reading the sentence in his turn in order to sign it, felt moved by pity for the poor wretch who had been condemned and, in the hope of obtaining some relaxation of his punishment, he came as close as he could to the ear of the auditor and said, pointing to Quasimodo:

'The man is deaf.'

He had hoped that this common infirmity would arouse Maître Florian's interest in favour of the prisoner. But in the first place, we have already observed that Maître Florian did not like it to be known he was deaf. And he was, secondly, so hard of hearing that he did not hear a single word of what the clerk was saying to him; however, he wanted to appear to have heard, and he answered: 'Ha, ha, that's different! I didn't know that. In that case, one hour extra in the pillory.'

And he signed the sentence so modified.

From *Notre-Dame de Paris*, translated by John Sturrock

Misfortune befalls the marriage of the Chevalier des Arcis and his young wife, Cecile.

The Chevalier des Arcis, an officer in the cavalry, had left the service in 1760. Although still young, and with means amply sufficient to allow him to appear to advantage at the Court, he had tired of bachelor's life and the pleasures of Paris. He retired to a pretty country house near Le Mans. Here, after a time, solitude, which had at first pleased him, became distasteful. He found that it was a difficult task to suddenly change from the habits of his youth. He did not repent having left the world of gaiety, but, not being able to live alone, he determined to marry and find, if possible, a woman with tastes similar to his own, and fond of the quiet and sedentary life that he had decided to live.

He did not wish his wife to be beautiful, nor did he want her ugly. He desired the woman he chose to be educated, intelligent, and not frivolous. What he wished for, above all, was cheerfulness and good disposition, which he regarded as being the first qualities a woman should possess.

The daughter of a retired merchant, who lived in the vicinity, pleased him. As the chevalier was not dependent upon any one, he did not worry about the social gap existing between a gentleman and a merchant's daughter. He asked the father for his daughter's hand, and the request was immediately acceded to. He courted her for a few months, and then they were married.

Never was a marriage celebrated under brighter and happier auspices. As he understood his wife better, the chevalier perceived in her new qualities and a uniform sweetness of disposition. She fell deeply in love with her husband. She lived but for him, thought only of pleasing him, and not regretting the pleasures that she had sacrificed at her age, she hoped that her whole existence might pass in this solitude, which daily became more precious to her . . .

The time fixed by nature at length arrived; a child, as beautiful as day, came into the world. It was a girl, whom they named Camille.

In spite of the general custom and even against the doctor's advice Cecile wished to nurse the little one herself. Her motherly pride was so flattered by the beauty of her daughter, that it was impossible to separate them. It is true that rarely in a new-born babe had such regular and such remarkable features been seen; its eyes, especially when they opened to the light, shone with wonderful lustre. Cecile, who had been raised in a convent, was extremely pious. Her first thought, as soon as she was able to be dressed, was to go to church to render thanks to God.

The child soon began to get strong and develop. As she grew they were astonished to find her unusually quiet. No noise seemed to disturb her; she was insensible to those thousand tender words that a mother addresses to her child; while she was being rocked and sung to, she would remain with fixed and open eyes, intently watching the light of the lamp, and seeming to hear nothing. One day, while asleep, a servant overturned a chair; her mother rushed up at once and noticed, with astonishment, that the child had not awakened. The chevalier became frightened at these indications, all too clear to be mistaken. As soon as he had carefully observed them, he understood to what misfortune his daughter was condemned. The mother wished in vain not to believe it, and by all imaginable means to turn away at her husband's fears. The physician was sent for, and his diagnosis was short and not difficult. They understood that poor Camille was deprived of the senses of hearing and speech.

The mother's first thought was to inquire if the misfortune was incurable, and the reply was that there had been a few cases which had been cured. For a year, in spite of the evidence, she continued to hope; but after having exhausted all the resources of science, they at length were compelled to abandon all hope.

Unfortunately, at this time, when so many prejudices were destroyed and replaced, there existed a most pitiless one against those poor creatures known as deaf-mutes . . . Everywhere, even in Paris, in the most advanced civilisation, deaf-mutes were looked upon as a kind of being separate from the rest of humanity, stamped with the seal of the wrath of Providence. Deprived of speech, they were given no credit for possessing the power of thought. The cloister for those who were born rich, abandonment or the poor; such was their lot. They inspired more horror than pity.

The chevalier gradually sank into the most profound melancholy. He spent the greater part of the day alone, shut up in his study or walking in the woods. When he saw his wife, he forced himself to appear tranquil and at rest, and attempted to console her, but without avail. Madame des Arcis was no less sad. A deserved misfortune may cause the tears to flow, usually too late and of no use; but a misfortune without reason benumbs the senses and discourages pity.

These two newly married people, made to love each other, in this way, commenced to see each other with pain and to avoid meeting in those same walks where they had so recently discussed a hope, so near, so peaceful, and so pure . . .

What caused this sudden and tacit separation, more terrible than a divorce, more cruel than slow death, was that the mother, in spite of the misfortune, loved her child passionately, while the chevalier, whatever he may have wished to do, in spite of his patience and goodness, could not conquer the horror that was inspired in him by this malediction of God that had fallen upon him . . .

Uncle Giraud, the master mason, did not think it such a misfortune that his niece was mute.

'I have had such a loquacious wife,' he would say, 'that I look upon anything in this world, whatever it may be, as preferable. This little girl is certain not to indulge in idle talk, nor listen to it, sure not to annoy the whole household by singing old opera airs, which are all alike; she will not be quarrelsome, she will not abuse the servants, as my wife always did; she will not awaken if her husband coughs, or if he arises before her in the morning to attend to his business. She will not dream aloud, but will be able to settle an account, even if she only counts on her fingers, and to pay, if she has the money, but without disputing, as do the merchants, over the least trifles. She will naturally know a very good thing, one which is ordinarily learned only with difficulty, and that is, that it is better to act than to talk. If her heart is in the right place, people will know it without it being necessary for her to put honey on the end of her tongue. She will not laugh in company, it is true; but, at dinner, she will not hear the foolish words spoken now and then. She will be pretty, intelligent and quiet; she will not be obliged like

the blind, to have a poodle to lead her. My faith! If I was young
would marry her myself, when she grows up; and today, now that
am old and childless, I will gladly take her as a daughter . . .'

From 'Pierre and Camille'*,
in Musset's *Contes*,
translated by Raoul Pelissie

* This classic of the fictional treatment of deafness has a happy ending
Camille, following Cecile's death, is brought up by Uncle Giraud, a
the chevalier rejects her. On a visit to Paris, Camille meets Pierre,
handsome marquis, deaf without speech like herself. They marry an
have a 'hearing' son. The story ends with Camille presenting he
child to the returning chevalier. The last words are Giraud's: 'Now
you see clearly that God pardons all, and always.'

What matters deafness of the ear, when
the mind hears. The one true deafness,
the incurable deafness, is that of the
mind.

Victor-Marie Hugo

Wemmick, Mr Jaggers' clerk, takes Pip to his home in Walworth, where he introduces him to his father.

I am my own engineer, and my own carpenter, and my own plumber, and my own gardener, and my own Jack of all Trades,' said Wemmick in acknowledging my compliments. 'Well, it's a good thing, you know. It brushes the Newgate cobwebs away, and pleases the Aged. You wouldn't mind being at once introduced to the Aged, would you? It wouldn't put you out?'

I expressed the readiness I felt, and we went into the castle. There, we found, sitting by a fire, a very old man in a flannel coat: clean, cheerful, comfortable, and well cared for, but intensely deaf.

'Well aged parent,' said Wemmick, shaking hands with him in a cordial and jocose way, 'how am you?'

'All right, John; all right!' replied the old man.

'Here's Mr Pip, aged parent,' said Wemmick, 'and I wish you could hear his name. Nod away at him, Mr Pip; that's what he likes. Nod away at him, if you please, like winking!'

'This is a fine place of my son's sir,' cried the old man, while I nodded as hard as I possibly could. 'This is a pretty pleasure-ground, sir. This spot and these beautiful works upon it ought to be kept together by the Nation, after my son's time, for the people's enjoyment.'

'You're as proud of it as Punch; ain't you, Aged?' said Wemmick, contemplating the old man, with his hard face really softened; '*there's* a nod for you;' giving him a tremendous one: '*there's* another for you;' giving him a still more tremendous one; 'you like that, don't you? If you're not tired, Mr Pip – though I know it's tiring for strangers – will you tip him one more? You can't think how it pleases him.'

I tipped him several more, and he was in great spirits.

From *Great Expectations*

99

Mr Pickwick meets Mr Wardle's mother at Dingley Dell.

A very old lady, in a lofty cap and faded silk gown – no less personage than Mr Wardle's mother – occupied the post of honou on the right-hand corner of the chimney-piece; . . . The aunt, th two young ladies, and Mr Wardle, each vying with the other i paying zealous and unremitting attentions to the old lady, crowde round her easy-chair, one holding her ear-trumpet, another a orange, and a third a smelling-bottle, while a fourth was busil engaged in patting and punching the pillows which were arrange for her support . . .

'Mr Pickwick, mother,' said Mr Wardle, at the very top of hi voice.

'Ah!' said the old lady, shaking her head; 'I can't hear you.'

'Mr Pickwick, grandma!' screamed both the young ladie together.

'Ah!' exclaimed the old lady. 'Well it don't much matter. He don' care for an old 'ooman like me, I dare say.'

'I assure you, ma'am,' said Mr Pickwick, grasping the old lady' hand, and speaking so loud that the exertion imparted a crimsor hue to his benevolent countenance, 'I assure you, ma'am, tha nothing delights me more than to see a lady of your time of lif heading so fine a family, and looking so young and well.'

'Ah!' said the old lady, after a short pause; 'it's all very fine, dare say; but I can't hear him.'

'Grandma's rather put out now,' said Miss Isabella Wardle, in low tone; 'but she will talk to you presently.'

Mr Pickwick nodded his readiness to humour the infirmities o age, and entered into a general conversation with the othe members of the circle.

From *The Posthumous Papers of the Pickwick Clul*

Miss Pross, on escaping with Mr Cruncher from the terror of the French Revolution, discovers that she has lost her hearing.

'Is there any noise in the streets?' she asked him.

'The usual noises,' Mr Cruncher replied; and looked surprised by the question and by her aspect.

'I don't hear you,' said Miss Pross. 'What do you say?'

It was in vain for Mr Cruncher to repeat what he said: Miss Pross could not hear him. 'So I'll nod my head,' thought Mr Cruncher, amazed, 'at all events she'll see that.' And she did.

'Is there any noise in the streets now?' asked Miss Pross again, presently.

Again Mr Cruncher nodded his head.

'I don't hear it.'

'Gone deaf in a hour?' said Mr Cruncher, ruminating, with his mind much disturbed: 'wot's come to her?'

'I feel,' said Miss Pross, 'as if there had been a flash and a crash,* and that crash was the last thing I should ever hear in this life.'

'Blest if she ain't in a queer condition!' said Mr Cruncher, more and more disturbed. 'Wot can she have been a takin', to keep her courage up? Hark! There's the roll of them dreadful carts! You can hear that, miss?'

'I can hear,' said Miss Pross, seeing that he spoke to her, 'nothing. O, my good man, there was first a great crash, and then a great stillness, and that stillness seems to be fixed and unchangeable, never to be broken any more as long as my life lasts.'

'If she don't hear the roll of those dreadful carts, now very nigh their journey's end,' said Mr Cruncher, glancing over his shoulder, 'it's my opinion that indeed she never will hear anything else in this world.'

And indeed she never did.

From A Tale of Two Cities

* A pistol shot, fired at close range, by Mme Defarge.

How 'Doctor' Marigold taught his 'adopted' daughter, who was deaf without speech.

You'd have laughed – or the rewerse – it's according to your disposition – if you could have seen me trying to teach Sophy. At first I was helped – you'd never guess by what – milestones. I got some large alphabets in a box, all the letters separate on bits of bone, and saying we was going to WINDSOR, I give her those letters in that order, and then at every milestone I showed her those same letters in that same order again, and pointed towards the abode of royalty. Another time I give her CART, and then chalked the same

101

upon the cart. Another time I give her DOCTOR MARIGOLD, and hung a corresponding inscription outside my waistcoat. People that met us might stare a bit and laugh, but what did I care, if she caught the idea? She caught it after long patience and trouble, and then we did begin to get on swimmingly, I believe you! At first she was a little given to consider me the cart, and the cart the abode of royalty, but that soon wore off. We had our signs, too, and they was hundreds in number . . .

This happiness went on in the cart till she was sixteen year old. By which time I began to feel not satisfied that I had done my whole duty by her, and to consider that she ought to have better teaching than I could give her. It drew a many tears on both sides when I commenced explaining my views to her; but what's right is right, and you can't neither by tears nor laughter do away with its character.

So I took her hand in mine, and I went with her one day to the Deaf and Dumb establishment in London, and when the gentleman come to speak to us, I says to him: 'Now, I'll tell you what I'll do with you, Sir. I am nothing but a Cheap Jack, but of late years I have laid by for a rainy day notwithstanding. This is my only daughter (adopted), and you can't produce a deafer nor a dumber. Teach her the most that can be taught her in the shortest separation that can be named, – state the figure for it, – and I am game to put the money down. I won't bate you a single farthing, Sir, but I'll put down the money here and now, and I'll thankfully throw you in a pound to take it. There!' The gentleman smiled, and then, 'Well, well,' says he, 'I must first know what she has learned already. How do you communicate with her?' Then I showed him, and she wrote in printed writing many names of things and so forth; and we held some sprightly conversation, Sophy and me, about a little story in a book which the gentleman showed her, and which she was able to read. 'This is most extraordinary,' says the gentleman; 'is it possible that you have been her only teacher?' 'I have been her only teacher, Sir,' I says, 'beside herself.' 'Then,' says the gentleman, and more acceptable words was never spoken to me, 'you're a clever fellow, and a good fellow.' This he makes known to Sophy, who kisses his hands, clasps her own, and laughs and cries upon it.

From 'Dr Marigold', in *Christmas Stories*

*A Muscovite widow, looked after by a household of serfs, orders the
removal of Mumu whose barking disturbs her sleep. Gerasim, the
deaf caretaker, whose inseparable companion the dog is, is allowed
to carry out the order himself.*

. . . the door of the little room opened, and Gerasim appeared. He
was wearing his best jacket and was leading Mumu by a string.
Eroshka stood aside and let him pass. Gerasim made for the gate.
The little boys and all who were in the yard followed him with their
eyes, in silence. He did not even turn round, and put on his cap
only when in the street. Gavrila sent Eroshka after him as an
observer. Eroshka saw from a distance that he went into an
eating-house together with the dog, and settled down to wait for
him to come out.

In the eating-house they knew Gerasim and understood his
signs. He ordered cabbage soup with meat and sat down leaning
his arms on the table. Mumu stood beside his chair, quietly looking
at him with her intelligent eyes. Her coat fairly shone: it was
evident that it was newly combed. They brought Gerasim the
cabbage soup. He crumbled bread into it, cut the meat up very
small, and put the plate on the floor. Mumu began to eat with her
usual good manners, hardly touching the food with her little snout.
Gerasim looked at her for a long time; two great tears suddenly
rolled from his eyes; one fell on the little dog's forehead, the second
into the cabbage soup. He covered his face with his hands. Mumu
ate up half the plateful and moved away licking her lips.

Gerasim got up, paid for the cabbage soup, and went out
followed by the somewhat puzzled glance of the waiter. Eroshka,
seeing Gerasim, jumped round a corner, and letting him pass,
again set off after him.

Gerasim walked without hurrying and did not let Mumu off the
string. Having reached the corner of the street, he stopped as if in
thought, and abruptly with rapid steps he made straight for the
Krimsky Brod. On the way he went into a yard of a house on to

which a wing was being built, and brought away from there two bricks under his arm. From the Krimsky Brod he turned off by the riverbank, went to a spot where, tied to stakes, were two little boats with oars (he had noticed them previously), and jumped into one of them with Mumu.

A lame old man came out from behind a hut standing at the corner of a vegetable-plot, and shouted after him. But Gerasim merely nodded his head and began to row so strongly, though against the stream, that in a trice he had covered upwards of two hundred yards. The old man stood there, for a while, scratched his back, first with his left, then with his right hand, and limped back to the hut.

And Gerasim rowed and rowed. Now Moscow was left behind. Now along the banks stretched meadows, market gardens, fields, groves of trees, peasants' huts came into sight. One felt the breath of the country. He dropped the oars, lowered his head to Mumu, who was sitting in front of him on a dry thwart – the bottom was covered with water – and he remained motionless, his powerful hands crossed over her back, the boat, meanwhile, being very slowly carried back towards the town by the flow of water. At last Gerasim sat upright; in haste and with a kind of pained anger on his face, wound the string about the bricks which he had taken, made a noose and put it round Mumu's neck, lifted her over the river, looked at her for the last time . . .

Trustingly and fearlessly she looked at him and gently wagged her tail. He turned away, shut his eyes, and opened his hands . . . Gerasim heard nothing – neither the sharp squeal of the falling Mumu, nor the heavy splash of the water; for him the noisiest day was still and silent as not the quietest night is silent for us, and when he opened his eyes again wavelets were hurrying, as before, along the river, as if chasing one another; as before they splashed and washed against the side of the boat, and only far behind him wide circles were moving on towards the bank.

From *Mumu*, translated by Jessie Domb and Zlata Shoenberg

Madonna, the 'deaf and dumb' heroine of Wilkie Collins's novel is introduced to the reader by the 'grotesquely shocking' description of her on a placard advertising the attractions of Jubber's Circus.

THE MYSTERIOUS FOUNDLING!

AGED TEN YEARS!!

TOTALLY DEAF AND DUMB!!!*

Mr Jubber, as proprietor of the renowned Circus, has the honour of informing the nobility, gentry, and public, that the above wonderful Deaf and Dumb Female Child will appear between the first and second parts of the evening's performances. Mr J has taken the liberty of entitling this Marvel of Nature, The Mysterious Foundling; no one knowing who her father is, and her mother having died soon after her birth, leaving her in charge of the Equestrian Company, who have been fond parents and careful guardians to her ever since.

She was originally celebrated in the annals of Jubber's Circus, or Eighth Wonder of the World, as The Hurricane Child of the Desert; having appeared in that character, whirled aloft at the age of seven years in the hand of Muley Ben Hassan, the renowned Scourer of Sahara, in his daring act of Equitation, as exhibited to the terror of all England, in Jubber's Circus. At that time she had her hearing and speech quite perfect. But Mr J deeply regrets to state that a terrific accident happened to her soon afterwards. Through no fault on the part of The Scourer (who, overcome by his feelings at the result of the above-mentioned frightful accident, has gone back to his native wilds a moody and broken-hearted man), she slipped from his hand while the three horses bestrode by the fiery but humane Arab were going at a gallop, and fell, shocking to relate, outside the Ring, on the boarded floor of the Circus. She was supposed to be dead. Mr Jubber instantly secured the inestimable assistance of the Faculty, who found that she was still alive, and set her arm, which had been broken. It was only afterwards discovered that she had utterly lost her sense of hearing. To use the emphatic language of the medical gentlemen (who all spoke with tears in their eyes), she had been struck stone deaf by the shock. Under those melancholy circumstances, it was found that the faculty of speech soon failed her altogether; and she is now therefore totally DEAF AND DUMB – but Mr J rejoices to say, quite cheerful and in good health notwithstanding.

Mr Jubber being himself the father of a family, ventures to think that these little particulars may prove of some interest to an Intelligent, a Sympathetic, and a Benevolent Public. He will simply allude, in conclusion, to the performances of the Mysterious Foundling, as exhibiting perfection hitherto unparalleled in the Art of Legerdemain, with wonders of untraceable intricacy on the cards, originally the result of abstruse calculations made by that renowned Algebraist, Mohammed Engedi, extending over a period of ten years, dating from the year 1215 of the Arab Chronology. More than this Mr Jubber will not venture to mention, for 'Seeing is Believing,' and the Mysterious Foundling must be seen to be believed. For prices of admission consult bottom of bill.

From *Hide and Seek*

---

* Collins's model for the 'lifelike' creation of his afflicted heroine was John Kitto's *Lost Senses* (see page 30).

Jim, a runaway slave, is haunted by an incident in his past.

I went to sleep, and Jim didn't call me when it was my turn. He often done that. When I waked up, just at day-break, he was setting there with his head down betwixt his knees, moaning and mourning to himself. I didn't take notice, nor let on. I knowed what it was about. He was thinking about his wife and his children, away up yonder, and he was low and homesick; because he hadn't ever been away from home before in his life; and I do believe he cared just as much for his people as white folks does for their'n. It don't seem natural, but I reckon it's so. He was often moaning and mourning that way, nights, when he judged I was asleep, and saying. 'Po' little 'Lizabeth! po' little Johnny! It's mighty hard; I spec' I ain't ever gwyne to see you no mo', no mo'!' He was a mighty good nigger, Jim was.

But this time I somehow got to talking to him about his wife and young ones; and by-and-by he says:

'What makes me feel so bad dis time, 'uz bekase I hear sumpn over yonger on de bank like a whack, er a slam, while ago, en it mine me er de time I treat my little 'Lizabeth so ornery. She warn't on'y 'bout fo' year ole, en she tuck de sk'yarlet-fever, en had a powerful rough spell; but she got well, en one day she was a-stannin' aroun', en I says to her, I says:

"Shet de do'".

She never done it; jis' stood dah, kiner smilin' up at me. It make me mad; en I says agin, mighty loud, I says:

"Doan' you hear me? – shet de do'!"

She jis' stood de same way, kiner smilin' up. I was a-bilin'! I says:

"I lay I *make* you mine!"

En wid dat I fetch' her a slap side de head dat sont her a-spralin'. Den I went into de yuther room, en 'uz gone 'bout ten minutes; en when I come back, dah was dat do' a s-stannin' open *yit*, en dat chile stannin' mos' right in it, a-lookin' down and mourning', en de

tears runnin' down. My, but I *wuz* mad, I was agwyne for de chile
but jis' den – it was a do' dat open innerds – jis' den, 'long come de
wind en slam it to, behine de chile, ker-*blam*! – en my lan', de chile
never move'! My breff mos' hop outer me; en I feel so – so – I doan
know *how* I feel. I crope out, all a-tremblin', en crope aroun' en
open de do' easy en slow, en poke my head in behind de chile, sof
en still, en all uv a sudden, I says *pow*! jis' as loud as I could yell: She
never budge! Oh, Huck, I bust out a-cryin' en grab her up in my
arms, en say, "Oh, de po' little thing! de Lord God Amighty fogive
po' ole Jim, kaze he never gwyne to fogive hisself as long's he live!"
Oh, she was plumb deef en dumb, Huck, plumb deef en dumb – en
I'd ben a-treat'n her so!'

From *The Adventures of Huckleberry Finn*

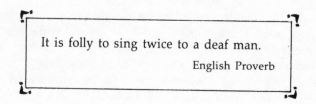

It is folly to sing twice to a deaf man.

English Proverb

The trumpet which didn't miss a word.

Did the hind, I wonder, with its beautiful trumpet ears, suggest the ear trumpet? Watching how this deer moved her pair of live trumpets about to catch passing sounds, it amused me to recall an old lady I used to see in a Hampshire village church who sat in a pew before mine during the Sunday morning services, and the deft way in which she manipulated her trumpet to capture the preacher's precious winged words. His manner of preaching was curious, if not quite unique. He would begin each sentence in a quiet natural tone, then raise his voice, then higher still, then let it drop back to the opening tone. Thus there were four changes in tone fitted to the four clauses composing each sentence, and there were also four bodily attitudes and movements to correspond. Thus the first clause was delivered standing in a stooping attitude, the eyes fixed on the MS [manuscript]. In the second he rose to his full height and fixed his eyes on his congregation. In the third the upward movement culminated in the preacher standing up on his toes, supporting himself by placing his finger-tips on the pulpit, and then having launched the words of clause three in his most powerful tones, he would sink back to the lower attitude, downward bent eyes and low voice. The difference in the man's height when he delivered clauses three and four must have been about nine inches, which would, of course, make a very great difference in listening to the sermon by a person hard of hearing. There the old lady's ear trumpet came in; there were four changes in its direction for each sentence, from the first and last when it was directed straight before her, to the second and third when it rose, automatically as it seemed, and at the third it would appear like a crest above her head.

I was told, if I remember rightly, that he had been vicar above a quarter of a century, and had always preached just in that way, and that the old lady had attended the church for many years with her ear trumpet, till long practice had made her so perfect in its use in following the sermon through all the preacher's bobbings up and down, she could almost do it with her eyes shut and never miss a word.

From *A Hind in Richmond Park*

The little boy has told on his brother. Uncle Remus disapproves and tells him the cautionary tale of 'The Fate of Mr Jack Sparrow'.

'W'at dat long rigmarole you bin tellin' Miss Sally 'bout yo' little brer dis mawnin?'

'Which, Uncle Remus?' asked the little boy, blushing guiltily.

'Dat des w'at I'm a axin' un you now. I hear Miss Sally say she's a gwineter stripe his jacket, en den I knowed you bin tellin' on 'im.'

'Well, Uncle Remus, he was pulling up your onions, and then he went and flung a rock at me,' said the child plaintively.

'Lemme tell you dis,' said the old man . . . 'der ain't no way fer ter make tattlers en tale-b'arers turn out good. No, dey ain't. I bin mixin' up wid fokes now gwine on eighty year, en I ain't seed no tattler come ter no good een'. Dat I ain't. En ef ole man M'thoozlum wuz livin' clean twel yit, he'd up'n tell you de same. Sho ez youer settin' dar. You 'member w'at 'com er de bird w'at went tattlin' 'roun' 'bout Brer Rabbit?'

The little boy didn't remember, but he was very anxious to know, and he also wanted to know what kind of a bird it was that so disgraced itself . . .

' "W'at dis twix' you en me, Brer Fox?" sez Brer Rabbit, sezee. "I hear tell you gwine ter sen' me ter 'struckshun, en nab my fambly, en 'stroy my shanty," sezee.

Den Brer Fox he git mighty mad.

"Who bin tellin' you all dis?" sezee.

Brer Rabbit make like he didn't want ter tell, but Brer Fox he 'sist en 'sist, twel at las' Brer Rabbit he up en tell Brer Fox dat he hear Jack Sparrer say all dis.

"Co'se," sez Brer Rabbit sezee, "w'en Brer Jack Sparrer tell me dat I flew up, I did, en I use some langwidge w'ich I'm mighty glad dey wern't no ladies 'roun' nowhars so dey could hear me go on," sezee.

Brer Fox he sorter gap, he did, en say he speck he better be sa'nter'n on. But, bless yo'soul, honey, Brer Fox ain't sa'nter fur, 'fo'

Jack Sparrer flipp down on a 'simmon-bush by de side er de road, en holler out:

"Brer Fox! Oh, Brer Fox! – Brer Fox."

Brer Fox he des sorter canter 'long, he did, en make like he don't hear 'im. Den Jack Sparrer up'n sing out agin:

"Brer Fox! Oh, Brer Fox! Hole on, Brer Fox! I got some news fer you. Wait, Brer Fox! Hit'll 'stonish you."

Brer Fox he make like he don't see Jack Sparrer, ner needer do he hear 'im, but bimeby he lay down by de road, en sorter stretch hisse'f like he fixin' for ter nap. De tattlin' Jack Sparrer he flew'd 'long, en keep on callin' Brer Fox, but Brer Fox, he ain't sayin' nuthin'. Den little Jack Sparrer, he hop down on de groun' en flutter 'roun 'mongst de trash. Dis sorter 'track Brer Fox 'tenshun, en he look at de tattlin' bird, en de bird he keep on callin':

"I got sump'n fer ter tell you, Brer Fox."

"Git on my tail, little Jack Sparrer," sez Brer Fox, sezee, "kaze I'm de'f in one year, en I can't hear out'n de udder. Git on my tail," sezee.

Den de little bird he up'n hop on Brer Fox's tail.

"Git on my back, little Jack Sparrer, kaze I'm de'f in one year en I can't hear out'n de udder."

Den de little bird hop on his back.

"Hop on my head, little Jack Sparrer, kaze I'm de'f in bofe years."

Up hop de little bird.

"Hop on my toof, little Jack Sparrer, 'kaze I'm de'f in one year en I can't hear out'n de udder."

De tattlin' little bird hop on Brer Fox's toof, en den — '

Here Uncle Remus paused, opened wide his mouth and closed it again in a way that told the whole story.

'Did the Fox eat the bird all – all – up?' asked the little boy.

'Jedge B'ar come 'long nex' day,' replied Uncle Remus, 'en he fine some fedders, en fum dat word went roun' dat ole man Squinch Owl done kotch mudder watz-izname.'

From *Uncle Remus: His Songs and His Sayings*

*The farmer Picot tells his neighbour the 'simple' story of Gargan,
the shepherd.*

But just as I emerged from the wood, I saw, standing ten paces
from me, Gargan, the deaf-mute, Monsieur Picot's herdsman,
wrapped round in a voluminous yellowish cloak, with a woollen
bonnet on his head, and knitting away at a stocking, as all the
shepherds of these parts do.

'Good morning, shepherd,' I said, as we always do.

And he lifted his head in greeting, although he had not heard my
voice, but he had seen my lips moving.

I have known this shepherd for fifteen years. For fifteen years I
have seen him every autumn, standing on the edge or in the
middle of a field, his body motionless and his hands ceaselessly
knitting. His flock follow him like a pack of hounds, seeming to
obey his eye.

Old Picot grasped my arm:

'You know that the shepherd has killed his wife?'

I was dumbfounded.

'Gargan? The deaf-mute?'

'Yes, this last winter, and he was brought to trial at Rouen. I will
tell you about it.'

And he drew me into the copse, for the herdsman was able to
pick up the words from his master's lips as if he had heard them.
He understood no one else; but face to face with him, he was no
longer deaf; and his master, on the other hand, read like a wizard
every meaning of the mute's dumb show, all the gestures of his
fingers, the wrinklings of his cheeks, and the flashes of his eyes.

Listen to this simple story, a melancholy piece of news, just such
a one as happens in the country, time and again.

Gargan was the son of a marl-digger, one of those men who go
down into the clay pits to dig out that sort of soft stone, white and
viscous, that we scatter on the fields. Deaf and dumb from birth, he
had been brought up to keep the cows along the roadside ditches.

112

Then, employed by Picot's father, he had become a shepherd at the farm. He was an excellent shepherd, zealous and honest, and he could set dislocated limbs, though he had not been taught anything of the kind.

When Picot came into the farm in his time, Gargan was thirty years old, and looked forty. He was tall, thin, and bearded, bearded like a patriarch.

Then, just about this time, Martel, an honest country woman, died, leaving a young girl of fifteen, who had been nicknamed 'A Wee Drop', because of her immoderate liking for brandy.

Picot took in this ragged young wretch and employed her in light tasks, feeding her without paying her wages, in return for her work. She slept in the barn, in the cattle-shed or in the stable, on straw or dung, any place, no matter where, for no one bothers to find a bed for these ragamuffins. She slept anywhere, with anyone, perhaps with the carter or the labourer. But it soon came about that she attached herself to the deaf-mute and formed a more lasting union with him. How did these two poor wretches come together? How did they understand each other? Had he ever known a woman before this barn rat, he who had never talked to a soul? Was it she who sought him out in his rolling hut and seduced him at the edge of the road, a hedge-side Eve? No one knows. It only became known one day, that they were living together as man and wife.

No one was surprised. And Picot even found this union quite natural.

But now the parish priest learned of this union without benefit of clergy, and was angry. He reproached Madame Picot, made her conscience uneasy, menaced her with mysterious penalties. What was to be done? It was quite simple. They were taken to the church and the town hall to be married. Neither of them had a penny to his name; he not a whole pair of trousers, she not a petticoat that was all of a piece. So nothing hindered the demands of State and Church from being satisfied. They were joined together, before mayor and priest, within one hour, and everything seemed arranged for the best.

But would you believe that, very soon, it became a joke in the country-side (forgive the scandalous word) to cuckold poor Gargan? Before the marriage, no one thought of lying with the Wee Drop; and now, everyone wanted his turn just for fun. For a brandy

113

she received all comers, behind her husband's back. The exploit was even so much talked of in the district round that gentlemen came from Goderville to see it.

Primed with a pint, the Wee Drop treated them to the spectacle with anyone, in a ditch, behind a wall, while at the same time the motionless figure of Gargan was in full view a hundred paces away, knitting a stocking and followed by his bleating flock. People laughed fit to kill themselves in all the inns in the country-side; in the evening, round the fire, nothing else was talked about; people hailed each other on the roads, asking: 'Have you given your drop to the Wee Drop?' Every one knew what that meant.

The shepherd seemed to see nothing. But then one day young Poirot from Sasseville beckoned Gargan's wife to come behind a haystack, letting her see a full bottle. She understood and ran to him, laughing; then, hardly were they well on the way with their evil work when the herdsman tumbled on them as if he had fallen from a cloud. Poirot fled, hopping on one leg, his trousers about his heels, while the mute, growling like a beast, seized his wife's throat.

People working on the common came running up. It was too late; her tongue was black and her eyes starting out of her head; blood was running out of her nose. She was dead.

The shepherd was tried by the Court at Rouen. As he was dumb, Picot served him as interpreter. The details of the affair were very amusing to the audience. But the farmer only had one idea, which was to get his herdsman acquitted, and he went about it very craftily.

He told them first the whole history of the deaf-mute and of his marriage; then, when he came to the crime, he himself cross-examined the murderer.

The whole Court was silent.

Picot said slowly:

'Did you know that she was deceiving you?'

And at the same time, he conveyed his question with his eyes. The other made a sign, 'no', with his head.

'She was lying in the haystack when you found her?'

And he gesticulated like a man who sees a revolting sight. The other made a sign, 'yes', with his head.

Then the farmer, imitating the gestures of the mayor performing the civil ceremony and of the priest uniting them in the name of God, asked his servant if he had killed his wife because she was joined to him before man and God.

The shepherd made a sign, 'yes', with his head.

Picot said to him:

'Now, show us how it happened.'

Then the deaf-mute himself acted the whole scene. He showed how he was sleeping in the haystack, how he had been awakened by feeling the movement of the straw, how he had looked round carefully, and had seen the thing.

He was standing stiffly between two policemen, and all at once he imitated the obscene actions of the criminal pair clasped together in front of him.

A great shout of laughter went up in the Court, then stopped dead; for the shepherd, his eyes wild, working his jaws and his great beard as if he had been gnawing something, his arms stretched out, his head thrust forward, repeated the ghastly gesture of a murderer strangling his victim.

And he howled horribly, so maddened with rage that he imagined himself still grasping her, and the policemen were forced to seize him and push him forcibly into a seat to quiet him.

A profound and agonised shudder ran through the Court. Then Farmer Picot, placing his hand on his servant's shoulder, said simply:

'He had his honour, this man before you.'

And the shepherd was acquitted.

> From 'The Deaf-Mute'*, in *The Complete Short Stories of Guy de Maupassant*

* De Maupassant features another deaf character in his story, 'Old Amable'.

Israel, the Jew, hero of Hall Caine's novel, seeks the salvation of his daughter Naomi, who was born blind and deaf.

Naomi knew nothing of God, having no way of speech with man. Would God condemn her for that, and cast her out for ever? No, no, no! God would not ask her for good works in the land of silence, and for labour in the land of night. She had no eyes to see God's beautiful world, and no ears to hear His holy word. God had created her so, and He would not destroy what He had made. Far rather would He look with love and pity on His little one, so long and sorely tried on earth, and send her at last to be a blessed saint in heaven.

Israel tried to comfort himself so, but the effort was vain . . .

Visions stood up before him of endless retribution for the soul that knew not God. These were the most awful terrors of his sleepless nights, but at length peace came to him, for he saw his path of duty. It was his duty to Naomi that he should tell her of God and reveal the word of the Lord to her! What matter if she could not hear? Though she had senses as the sands of the seashore, yet in the way of light the Lord alone could lead her. What matter though she could not see? The soul was the eye that saw God, and with bodily eyes had no man seen Him.

So every day thereafter at sunset Israel took Naomi by the hand and led her to an upper room, the same wherein her mother died, and, fetching from a cupboard on the wall the Book of the Law, he read to her of the commandments of the Lord by Moses, and of the Prophets, and of the Kings. And while he read Naomi sat in silence at his feet, with his one free hand in both of her hands, clasped close against her cheek.

What the little maid in her darkness thought of this custom, what mystery it was to her and wherefore, only the eye that looks into darkness could see; but it was so at length that as soon as the sun had set – for she knew when the sun was gone – Naomi herself would take her father by the hand, and lead him to the upper room, and fetch the book to his knees.

116

And sometimes, as Israel read, an evil spirit would seem to come to him, and make a mock at him, and say, 'The child is deaf and hears not – go read your book in the tombs!' But he only hardened his neck and laughed proudly. And, again, sometimes the evil spirit seemed to say, 'Why waste yourself in this misspent desire? The child is buried while she is still alive, and who shall roll away the stone?' But Israel only answered, 'It is for the Lord to do miracles, and the Lord is mighty.'

So, great in his faith, Israel read to Naomi night after night, and when his spirit was sore of many taunts in the day his voice would be hoarse, and he would read the law which says. *'Thou shalt not curse the deaf, nor put a stumbling-block before the blind.'* But when his heart was at peace his voice would be soft, and he would read of the child Samuel sanctified to the Lord in the temple, and how the Lord called him and he answered –

'And it came to pass at that time, when Eli was laid down in his place, and his eyes began to wax dim, that he could not see; and ere the lamp of God went out in the temple of the Lord, where the Ark of God was, and Samuel was laid down to sleep, that the Lord called Samuel, and he answered, Here am I. And he ran unto Eli and said, Here am I, for thou calledst me. And he said, I called not; lie down again. And he went and lay down. And the Lord called yet again, Samuel. And Samuel rose and went to Eli and said, Here am I, for thou didst call me. And he answered, I called not, my son; lie down again. Now Samuel did not yet know the Lord, neither was the word of the Lord yet revealed to him.'

And, having finished his reading, Israel would close the book, and sing out of the Psalms of David the psalm which says, *'It is good for me that I have been in trouble, that I may learn Thy statutes.'*

Thus, night after night, when the sun was gone down, did Israel read of the law and sing of the Psalms to Naomi, his daughter, who was both blind and deaf. And though Naomi heard not, and neither did she see, yet in their silent hour together there was another in their chamber always with them – there was a third, for there was God.

From *The Scapegoat*

The landlady's story.

I was born at Yarmouth, though it is many and many a year since
have seen a herringboat. You see, my story is a very simple one.
was an orphan girl, for my dear father was drowned in an Octobe
gale when fishing at sea, and I came to London with a family a
nursemaid. They did not treat me kindly – even now I cannot sa
that they did, although I wish to be charitable – for they discharge
me because I was not strong enough to do the work, and if I had no
been taken in out of pity by a widow woman, a dressmaker and m
predecessor in this very house, I do not know what would hav
become of me.

My husband was her only child, and it was part of my duty, an
indeed of my pleasure, to look after him in his affliction* so far as
was able. Then when his mother died I married him, for I could no
make up my mind to leave him alone, and this of course I mus
have done unless I became his wife. So you see, my dear, I took hin
on and the business with him, and we have been very happy eve
since – so happy that I sometimes wonder why God is so good t
me, who am full of faults. One sorrow we have had, it is true
though now even that seems to have become a joy: it was after Sall
was born. She was a beautiful baby, and when for the first time
grew sure that she would be deaf and dumb also, I cried till
thought my heart would break, and wished that she might die
Now I see how wicked that was, and every night I thank Heaves
that I was not taken at my word, for then my heart would hav
broken indeed.

From *Joan Hast*

* He was paralytic as well as deaf without speech.

Razumov's revelation that he had been responsible for the capture and execution of Victor Haldin, the famous revolutionary, leads to a swift and brutal revenge.

He turned his back on the room, and walked towards the stairs, but, at the violent crash of the door behind him, he looked over his shoulder and saw that Nikita, with three others, had followed him out. 'They are going to kill me, after all,' he thought.

Before he had time to turn round and confront them fairly, they set on him with a rush. He was driven headlong against the wall. 'I wonder how,' he completed his thought. Nikita cried, with a shrill laugh right in his face, 'We shall make you harmless. You wait a bit.'

Razumov did not struggle. The three men held him pinned against the wall, while Nikita, taking up a position a little on one side, deliberately swung off his enormous arm. Razumov, looking for a knife in his hand, saw it come at him open, unarmed, and received a tremendous blow on the side of his head over his ear. At the same time he heard a faint, dull detonating sound, as if someone had fired a pistol on the other side of the wall. A raging fury awoke in him at this outrage. The people in Laspara's rooms, holding their breath, listened to the desperate scuffling of four men all over the landing; thuds against the walls, a terrible crash against the very door, then all of them went down together with a violence which seemed to shake the whole house. Razumov, overpowered, breathless, crushed under the weight of his assailants, saw the monstrous Nikita squatting on his heels near his head, while the others held him down, kneeling on his chest, gripping his throat, lying across his legs.

'Turn his face the other way,' the paunchy terrorist directed, in an excited, gleeful squeak.

Razumov could struggle no longer. He was exhausted; he had to watch passively the heavy open hand of the brute descend again in a degrading blow over his other ear. It seemed to split his head in two, and all at once the men holding him became perfectly silent soundless as shadows. In silence they pulled him brutally to h feet, rushed with him noiselessly down the staircase, and, openin the door, flung him out into the street.

He fell forward, and at once rolled over and over helplessly going down the short slope together with the rush of running rai water. He came to rest in the roadway of the street at the bottom lying on his back, with a great flash of lightning over his face – vivid, silent flash of lightning which blinded him utterly. H picked himself up, and put his arm over his eyes to recover h sight. Not a sound reached him from anywhere, and he began t walk, staggering, down a long, empty street. The lightning wave and darted round him its silent flames, the water of the deluge fel ran, leaped, drove – noiseless like the drift of mist. In this unearthl stillness his footsteps fell silent on the pavement, while a dum wind drove him on and on, like a lost mortal in a phantom worl ravaged by a soundless thunderstorm. God only knows where h noiseless feet took him to that night, here and there, and back agai without pause or rest. Of one place, at least, where they did lea him, we heard afterwards; and, in the morning, the driver of th first south-shore tramcar, clanging his bell desperately, saw bedraggled, soaked man without a hat, and walking in the roadwa unsteadily with his head down, step right in front of his car, and g under.

When they picked him up, with two broken limbs and a crushe side, Razumov had not lost consciousness. It was as though he ha tumbled, smashing himself, into a world of mutes. Silent mer moving unheard, lifted him up, laid him on the sidewalk, gesticu lating and grimacing round him their alarm, horror, and compas sion. A red face with moustaches stooped close over him, lip moving, eyes rolling, Razumov tried hard to understand the reaso of this dumb show. To those who stood around him, the features c that stranger, so grievously hurt, seemed composed in meditatior Afterwards his eyes sent out at them a look of fear and close slowly. They stared at him. Razumov made an effort to remembe some French words.

'Je suis sourd,' he had time to utter feebly, before he fainted.

'He is deaf,' they exclaimed to each other. 'That's why he did n hear the car.'

They carried him off in that same car . . .

. . . hours before, while the thunderstorm still raged in the night, there had been in the rooms of Julius Laspara a great sensation. The terrible Nikita, coming in from the landing, uplifted his squeaky voice in horrible glee before all the company –

'Razumov! Mr Razumov! The wonderful Razumov! He shall never be any use as a spy on any one. He won't talk, because he will never hear anything in his life – not a thing! I have burst the drums of his ears for him. Oh, you may trust me. I know the trick. Ha! Ha! Ha! I know the trick.'

From *Under Western Eyes*

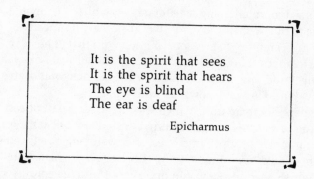

It is the spirit that sees
It is the spirit that hears
The eye is blind
The ear is deaf

Epicharmus

The story of Luney Joe.

Candleford Green had its village idiot in the form of a young man who had been born a deaf mute. At birth he was probably not mentally deficient, but he had been born too early to profit by the marvellous modern system of training such unfortunates, and had, as a child, been allowed to run wild while other children were in school, and the isolation and the absence of all means of communicating with his fellows had told upon him.

At the time when Laura knew him, he was a full-grown man, powerfully built, with a small golden beard his mother kept clipped and, in his quieter moments, an innocent rather than a vacant expression. His mother, who was a widow, took in washing and he would fetch and carry her clothes-baskets, draw water from the well, and turn the handle of the mangle. At home the two of them used a rough language of signs which his mother had invented, but with the outside world he had no means of communication and, for that reason, coupled with that of his occasional fits of temper, although he was strong and probably capable of learning to do any simple manual work, no one would give him employment. He was known as Luney Joe.

Joe spent his spare time, which was the greater part of each day, lounging about the green, watching the men at work at the forge or in the carpenter's shop. Sometimes, after watching quietly for some time, he would burst into loud inarticulate cries which were taken for laughter, then turn and run quickly out into the country where he had many lairs in the woods and hedgerows. Then the men would laugh and say: 'Old Luney Joe's like the monkeys. They could talk if they'd a mind to, but they think if they did we'd set 'em to work.'

If he got in the way of the workmen, they would take him by the shoulders and run him outside, and it was chiefly his wild gestures, contortions of feature, and loud inarticulate cries at such times which had earned him his name.

'Luney Joe! Luney Joe!' the children would call out after him, secure in the knowledge that, whatever they said, he could not hear them. But, although he was deaf and dumb, Joe was not blind, and once or twice, when he had happened to look round and see them following and mocking him, he had threatened them by shaking the ash stick he carried. The story of this lost nothing in the telling, and people were soon saying that Joe was getting dangerous and ought to be put away. But his mother fought stoutly for his liberty, and the doctor supported her. Joseph was sane enough, he said; his seeming strangeness came from his affliction. Those against him would do well to see that their own children were better behaved.

What went on in Joe's mind nobody knew, though his mother, who loved him, may have had some idea. Laura many times saw him standing to gaze on the green with knitted brows, as though puzzling as to why other young men should be batting and bowling there and himself left out. Once some men unloading logs to add to Miss Lane's winter store allowed Joe to hand down from the cart some of the heaviest, and, for a time, his face wore an expression of perfect happiness. After a while, unfortunately, his spirits soared and he began flinging the logs down wildly and, as a result, hit one of the men on the shoulder, and was turned away roughly. At that, he fell into one of his passions and, afterwards, people said that Luney Joe was madder than ever.

But he could be very gentle. Once Laura met him in a lonely spot between trees and she felt afraid, for the path was narrow and she was alone. But she felt ashamed of her cowardice afterwards, for, as she passed him, so closely that their elbows touched, the big fellow, gentle as a lamb, put out his hand and stroked some flowers she was carrying. With nods and smiles, Laura passed on, rather hurriedly, it must be confessed, but wishing more than ever she could do something to help him.

Some years after Laura had left the district she was told that, after his mother's death, Luney Joe had been sent to the County Asylum. Poor Joe! the world which went very well for some people in those days was a harsh one for the poor and afflicted.

From *Candleford Green*

Mrs Stratton and her son Gilbert see the headmaster on Gilbert's first day at a school for the deaf.

The child – he was only seven – stood silent, lonely, passive, patient, with eyes apparently looking vacantly at the opposite wall, as deaf children will when others are talking of them. For though they hear nothing they know perfectly well when the conversation is about themselves.

And Gilbert Stratton waited while the mother who loved but did not understand him, and the headmaster who did not love as much but did understand better, conversed together; waited in an office surrounded with maps that were unintelligible, books that were meaningless, figures that conveyed nothing, while people spoke words which were inaudible to him and which would have been incomprehensible even if audible; waited, as the deaf always have waited, but will not have to wait much longer, perhaps.

Lonely he had always been, lonely with an intensity of loneliness utterly unknown to those around him and unrealised even by his parents. But he had accepted it as the deaf accept all their trials, and they are many. It was part of his lot.

But suddenly, as he still stood apparently looking at nothing, he saw the door slowly open and a boy a year younger than himself quietly enter. He walked aimlessly, as it seemed, with head down and hands behind him, in that shy way which children of six have when they wish to be unnoticed. Pausing when opposite to Gilbert on the other side of the room, he remained with head averted till he knew the cursory glances of the seniors present were no longer directed towards him, and then he cautiously raised his eyes and fixed them on the deaf boy's face.

The latter saw it all, and as soon as he felt that he was unobserved by anyone else he allowed his glance to meet that of the other. In an instant the younger, with enquiry stamped on every feature, flicked his right index finger to his ear, then to his mouth, and then pointed at the deaf boy, asking, as plainly as words could say it, 'Are you deaf and dumb?'

Utterly taken aback at being addressed in the only method of communication he understood, Gilbert nodded, open-eyed.

With a smile the other again pointed to ear and mouth, and then, alternately clenching his fists and opening his hands with fingers extended several times, and finally pointing through the door, conveyed the news that there were many more deaf and dumb in another room beyond.

Mrs Stratton at that moment turned her head, and instantly the faces of both boys were as impassive as blocks of marble.

For a few minutes Gilbert remained thus gazing straight in front of him. But the delight of the sudden revelation that there was someone here who talked in a language he could comprehend, the language of natural gesture, and that there were many more in that same house who were deaf – deaf like himself – surged with such force through his bewildered brain that his lip quivered. It meant – nay, what did it not mean to him? There were boys and girls in that house who could sympathise, could literally feel as he did, who had passed through what he had passed through, who had seen persons come up to them and look at them curiously and turn to others and mouth inaudibly about them, who had seen their own mothers sorrowfully join in the talk about them, who had had doctors prying and peering into their ears and nose and mouth, and talking, unheard by them, to their fathers about it all, but who had never found anyone to tell them what all the talk was about, had never met anyone who had ever shown any suspicion that they, poor children, could feel any pain at being examined and discussed and kept in ignorance as to what it all meant. There were children there who had experienced all this just as he had, who knew what he knew – the sensitiveness, the shame, the loneliness which was almost intensified by his own parents' attitude. For his love for his father and mother, and their love for him, made their failure to understand and sympathise all the harder to bear.

He was no longer alone! His head swam and he bit his lip. The long and bitter training of past years had made him outwardly unemotional, but the pent-up feelings within him refused to be suppressed. His lips quivered and quivered again; his frame shook. He clenched his hands tightly in an unconscious pride and rebellion against showing these strangely uncomprehending people what he felt, but the strength of his emotion was too great.

He suddenly buried his burning face in his hands and burst in tears.

'Poor boy!' exclaimed Mrs Stratton, as she took him into embrace; 'he feels the parting from us.'

Which was perfectly true, of course. But which was not the wh truth.

Mr Gordon quietly went on reading the form before hi Unknown to the two children he had seen their brief conversati out of the corner of his eye, and he understood what Mrs Stratt did not. For he was deaf himself, and had passed all but the first t years of his life among the deaf.

From *King Sile*

> The same battle in the clouds will be known to the deaf only as lightning and to the blind only as thunder.
>
> George Santayana

Bertha Coombe, a distant relative, lives with Mrs Meryon and her daughter Laura. In their presence, Mrs Meryon tells Mrs Edwards, a visitor, one of 'the most horrible stories'.

It's one of the most horrible stories,' said Mrs Meryon. 'I was really quite afraid to have her here, in case the sight of her should perpetually remind me of it. Her mother practically killed her father.'

'Killed! Do you mean it? And she doesn't know? Oh, but take care then!' whispered Mrs Edwards, her scruples aroused once more.

'It's quite all right, she can't hear a word. I'll tell you the whole story –'

'Here? Now?' asked Mrs Edwards, still half uneasy.

'Why not? We're talking about the *soufflé* we had at lunch, or about my new costume, for all she knows. Or – look! I'm showing you something highly interesting in my book,' she said, unable to repress a smile at her idea. She leaned over, and with great over-emphasis pretended to be showing her friend something in the book that was still in her hand.

'Well,' she resumed, 'Bertha was a child away at school when it happened. Her mother was deaf – as deaf as she is. She had become so gradually, just as Bertha has done. The father was my cousin, and a most charming man. Being very good-looking and popular, you can imagine what a drag on him his wife must have been, especially as she was madly devoted to him. They lived in a tiny old-fashioned house in Chelsea. Their maid fell ill and went to hospital; and Leslie, my cousin, so as to be out of the way of the discomfort and upset, was to go and stay for a few days with some friends. On the day he was to go, his wife suddenly found him disappeared. She thought he had gone without saying good-bye, as he sometimes did after a quarrel, and she admitted that there had been a scene that morning. But do you know what had happened really?'

'Mother! Stop!' implored Laura silently.

Bertha made a little hopeful movement. Such entranced glance – Surely this must be something she would be told. But howev urgent and important it might seem, she must not ask – she h. learnt that. People never liked it. Something was interesting the rushing through their minds at its own pace, and they never lik it if everything had to be stopped and brought to a standstill wh they communicated it to her. The only hope was to discover lat though how rarely this succeeded! – for people were general unable to recall what they had been speaking of, even though had looked on their faces at the time almost as if it must be a matt of life and death to them.

'What happened really,' Mrs Meryon went on, 'was that just he was ready to go, my cousin went to fetch a bottle of his spec wine to take with him. It was kept in a large, dark closet that led o of the sitting-room down two or three steps. While he was there tl door must have blown shut and, as it slammed, the outside bolt f and he was fastened in.

'All that day, and the days that followed, his wife was sitting that room, eating, reading, amusing herself, while a few yar away from her he was shouting and knocking and struggling f his life. He must have heard every movement of hers, just the oth side of the door, but however much he might shout she just calm went on with what she was doing, and let the husband she w supposed to love call and shout to her to save his life!'

'You mean she couldn't hear?' her friend broke in.

'Not a sound! Only you'd think some instinct might have to her, considering he was only two or three feet away from her. Late when he was missed, a search was made and he was found, but I died of exhaustion as they picked him up. When his wife kne what she had done she got into such a state that no one could anything for her. She couldn't get over it. The thought of it mu have haunted her day and night. She hardly spoke, and she nev seemed more than half alive after that. I used to see her sometime but she died a few years later. Her closest relations decided th Bertha should never be told what had happened. She was growir deaf herself, and they thought it might prey on her mind. They m; have decided rightly – I don't know.'

Bertha Coombe looked from one to the other in her docil inevitable patience. No, she must not interrupt and ask them –

did not do. And yet could she not ask Laura? With one who was so willing and responsive it was different, it was possible. Laura had a way of seeming even pleased to be put to some little trouble. As unnoticeably as possible, Bertha spoke to her:

'What is it they are saying? Something very interesting, I know! I couldn't quite hear. What are they talking about, dear?'

'We were just saying,' began Laura, bending down, 'we were just saying . . .'

From 'We Were Just Saying . . .', in *Young Mrs Cruse*

Naught shall the psaltry and the harp
   avail,
The pleasing song, or well repeated tale,
When the quick spirits their warm march
   forbear,
And numbing coldness has unbraced the
   ear.

Matthew Prior

Shortly before his death, Colonel Pinner meets Cyril, his grandson, for the last time.

They knocked at the door, and Cyril followed his aunts into grandfather's hot sweetish room.

'Come on,' said Grandfather Pinner. 'Don't hang about. What is it? What've you been up to?'

He was sitting in front of a roaring fire, clasping his stick. He had a thick rug over his knees. On his lap there lay a beautiful pale yellow silk handkerchief.

'It's Cyril, father,' said Josephine shyly. And she took Cyril's hand and led him forward.

'Good afternoon, grandfather,' said Cyril, trying to take his hand out of Aunt Josephine's. Grandfather Pinner shot his eyes at Cyril in the way he was famous for. Where was Auntie Con? She stood on the other side of Aunt Josephine; her long arms hung down in front of her; her hands were clasped. She never took her eyes off grandfather.

'Well,' said Grandfather Pinner, beginning to thump, 'what have you got to tell me?'

What had he, what had he got to tell him? Cyril felt himself smiling like a perfect imbecile. The room was stifling, too.

But Aunt Josephine came to his rescue. She cried brightly, 'Cyril says his father is still very fond of meringues, father dear.'

'Eh?' said Grandfather Pinner, curving his hand like a purple meringue-shell over one ear.

Josephine repeated, 'Cyril says his father is still very fond of meringues.'

'Can't hear,' said old Colonel Pinner. And he waved Josephine away with his stick, then pointed with his stick to Cyril. 'Tell me what she's trying to say,' he said.

(My God!) 'Must I?' said Cyril, blushing and staring at Aunt Josephine.

'Do, dear,' she smiled. 'It will please him so much.'

'Come on, out with it!' cried Colonel Pinner testily, beginning to thump again.

And Cyril leaned forward and yelled, 'Father's still very fond of meringues.'

At that Grandfather Pinner jumped as though he had been shot.

'Don't shout!' he cried. 'What's the matter with the boy? *Meringues*! What about 'em?'

'Oh, Aunt Josephine, must we go on?' groaned Cyril desperately.

'It's quite all right, dear boy,' said Aunt Josephine, as though he and she were at the dentist's together. 'He'll understand in a minute.' And she whispered to Cyril, 'He's getting a bit deaf, you know.' Then she leaned forward and really bawled at Grandfather Pinner, 'Cyril only wanted to tell you, father, dear, that *his* father is still very fond of meringues.'

Colonel Pinner heard that time, heard and brooded, looking Cyril up and down.

'What an esstrordinary thing!' said old Grandfather Pinner. 'What an esstrordinary thing to come all this way here to tell me!'

And Cyril felt it *was*.

'Yes, I shall send Cyril the watch,' said Josephine.

'That would be very nice,' said Constantia.

From 'The Daughters of the Late Colonel', in *The Garden Party*

*Timmy Tiverton, an elderly music-hall artist, visits 'Packles',
theatrical agents, in search of employment.*

'Packles' were at the back of one of the larger and dirtier houses in
Shelving square, and Timmy succeeded at once in seeing young Mr
Packles, who had a swollen face.

'It's a gumboil,' he explained gloomily. 'Hurts like hell. Didn't
get a wink o' sleep last night.'

'Sorry to hear that.' And Timmy was, very sorry.

Young Mr Packles, who was not very young, grunted. 'Well, I 've
'eard of you, of course—'

'Of course,' cried Timmy cheerfully and confidently. 'Top o' the
bill—'

'But it's a long time since,' young Packles continued brutally.
'About when I was still at school. If I'd been asked, I'd 'ave said you
were dead an' buried.' . . .

'We like bang-up-to-date acts.' And Mr Packles waved his hand,
though at what, Timmy could not imagine. 'B.B.C. turns, specially,
I don't think you've been on the air, 'ave you?'

'No,' replied Timmy, who had faced this awkward question
before and hated it like poison. 'I like my public to see me.'

'He wants *what?*' This question came in a shout from about
twelve inches behind Timmy's ear. He jumped, then turned
indignantly. An elderly man, with a long spreading kind of nose
and suspicious little eyes too close together at the top of it, was
standing there, bending forward and holding a black ear-trumpet
almost big enough for a gramophone.

'He says, Dad, he likes 'is public to see 'im,' bellowed young Mr
Packles.

'What public?' shouted Mr Packles, moving his trumpet round
from his son to Timmy.

'Any public,' roared Timmy, almost inside the trumpet.

Old Mr Packles nodded, as if somehow all this confirmed his
worst suspicions, then said quietly to his son: 'I don't catch on to

all this, Fred, but if he wants an audition, he can 'ave one.' He turned to Timmy again. 'Comedian, eh?'

'That's right,' Timmy shouted. 'Comedian. Funny man. Make you laugh.'

'You come into the other room then, an' make us laugh. Eh, Fred? How's your face this morning? Looks a lot worse to me.'

'An' it feels a lot worse,' his son told him gloomily. 'This way, Mr What's-it' . . .

'If you want a pianist,' said young Mr Packles, 'You'll have to wait till this afternoon.'

'I can manage,' said Timmy grimly. 'Of course, you're not seeing the act under the best conditions. I mean to say—'

'That's all right. We're used to it.'

'We've 'ad some of the best 'ere, the very best,' old Mr Packles shouted in his startling tuneless voice. 'You go on. Make us laugh.'

Timmy nodded, closed his eyes a second, tried to forget he was in a backroom on Monday morning in Birchester with this awful pair, then all desperate comic sparkle, he began one of his favourite numbers. 'Now the missis once moved in socie-tee,' he sang, loudly and confidently, but feeling like one of the front rank of the Light Brigade. He did one verse and the chorus, then went into his patter. 'You don't know my wife, do you?' he asked the Packles, who were now looking as if they had never known anybody. 'My wife's a very fine woman, a very fine woman. Very fond of pets. I'll never forget the time she came back with a bird-cage. "Look at what I've got," she says. "Well, Maria, what've you got?" I asks. "It's a parrot," she says—'

'Half a minute,' young Mr Packles interrupted gloomily. 'Is this the one about the parrot that didn't like cheese?'

'That's right,' replied Timmy, feeling like a burst balloon. 'I always find it gets a big laugh – the way I tell it.'

'We know it. Dad,' he shouted down the trumpet, 'it's the one about the parrot that didn't like cheese. I'm telling 'im we know it.'

'Quite right,' said his father, in what he mistakenly thought a whisper. 'Doesn't seem to 'ave much go about 'im, this chap, does he? But we'll give 'im another two or three minutes.'

Timmy swallowed hard, told himself to remember that this seemed about his last chance, then plunged into his patter again. 'And then there's my brother. What a man! I say, what a man! I'll never forget the day he got married. Now we all went along early in the morning—'

It was here that old Mr Packles leaned towards his son and spoke again in what he imagined to be a whisper, completely drowning Timmy. 'I told your mother to stop in bed to-day,' said old Mr Packles. 'I told her if she didn't rest properly to-day, with her legs in that state again, she'll 'ave another fortnight of it, an' a nurse into the bargain.' Then he turned, rather startled, towards Timmy. 'What did you say?'

'I said *good morning*,' Timmy shouted at the top of his voice. 'You lot don't want a comic, you want a clinic.'

From *Let the People Sing*

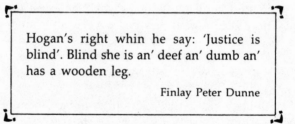

Hogan's right whin he say: 'Justice is blind'. Blind she is an' deef an' dumb an' has a wooden leg.

Finlay Peter Dunne

El Sordo (the Deaf One) guerrilla leader on the Republican side during the Spanish Civil War, welcomes Pilar, another guerrilla leader and Robert Jordan, the American 'dynamiter' to his camp.

El Sordo was short and heavy, brown-faced, with broad cheekbones; grey haired, with wide-set yellow-brown eyes, a thin-bridged, hooked nose like an Indian's, a long upper lip and a wide, thin mouth. He was clean shaven and he walked toward them from the mouth of the cave, moving with the bow-legged walk that went with his cattle herdsman's breeches and boots. The day was warm but he had on a sheep's wool-lined short leather jacket buttoned up to the neck. He put out a big brown hand to Pilar. '*Hola*, woman' he said. '*Hola*' he said to Robert Jordan and shook his hand and looked him keenly in the face. Robert Jordan saw his eyes were yellow as a cat's and flat as a reptile's eyes are . . .

'Where do you get the whisky?'

'What?' he could not hear.

'You have to shout,' Pilar said. 'Into the other ear.'

El Sordo pointed to his better ear and grinned.

'Where do you get the whisky?' Robert Jordan shouted.

'Make it,' El Sordo said and watched Robert Jordan's hand check on its way to his mouth with the glass.

'No,' El Sordo said and patted his shoulder. 'Joke. Comes from La Granja. Heard last night comes English dynamiter. Good. Very happy. Get whisky. For you. You like?'

'Very much,' said Robert Jordan. 'It's very good whisky.'

'Am contented,' Sordo grinned . . .

From *For Whom the Bell Tolls*

135

On her return from America millionairess Eva Trout visits old friends. Henry has already discovered that her 'adopted' son, Jeremy, is deaf without speech, but Henry's father, Mr Dancey, has still to be told.

Mr Dancey brought Jeremy into focus. 'And who's this?' he said – not without apprehension. Eva replied by advancing Jeremy, beautifully – the child looked mildly up at the clergyman. Eva said to him: 'This is Mr Dancey.' The two shook hands. 'First visit to England?' asked Mr Dancey. Jeremy smiled.

'In a manner of speaking,' said Henry, 'her little boy.'

'Mr Dancey,' said Eva, argumentatively, stoutly, and yet beseechingly, 'there's nothing wrong about Jeremy.'

'Nothing,' he said, regarding the child with pleasure, 'that I can see. – Henry, what about tea?' ... And all this time you've been where? Did I hear, America?'

'Yes. We . . .'

'Then I do truly envy you. An exciting, I imagine an endless country. Here, we—'

'I am going,' cut in Henry, 'to boil the kettle. Eva, better tell Father, or there'll be bother later.'

'I dislike,' Mr Dancey said, 'being talked across. I am not yet senile.' Henry went to the kitchen. 'What did he mean, though?' went on his father. 'What am I to be told?' Jeremy made a diversion by towing Mr Dancey to the hearthrug, to admire the masterpiece.* 'He's clever,' guaranteed Eva, following after. 'Only, what Henry meant is, he does not hear and does not speak.'

The startled man said: 'I should never have known.' He looked the more intently down at the pattern. 'Sight to me is the thing – the thing above all things. And more seeing eyes than his I have seldom seen. And they must be, or he couldn't have made this.' Mr Dancey, spotting a fragment of Crown Derby, ejaculated: 'The last of a wedding present! Twelve of everything, inconceivable now! . . . But surely, Eva,' he said most earnestly, 'in these days, and in

136

that progressive country you've been in, something could have been done, has been done: what is being done?'

'Everything! – that is to say, very, very, much.' Eva spoke with a passion that yet had somewhere in it a hint of evasion. 'But Jeremy doesn't like it; he doesn't want to. He not only doesn't co-operate, they all tell me, he puts a resistance up. He is angered by what they attempt to do to him. It upsets him. He would like to stay happy the way he is.'

'Many of us would; but that's not the thing. – Oh come, Eva, who would not wish to speak?'

'I have never wished to. What is the object? What is the good?'

'Or, hear?' he continued – changing his ground. 'Crass as sound can be, imagine a soundless world! No, this child has come into your life, however he did, and you must *not* doom him. I do mean "doom"; you doom if you acquiesce. You dare not,' he added, abating the verb a little by his compassion. 'There cannot – somewhere? – be someone who cannot help, cannot handle him. I cannot believe you have yet tried everything: try everything! Search Europe.'

From *Eva Trout*

* A pattern made of oddments, accumulated by Jeremy.

The kindness of Robinson, owner of 'Bellevue', revives in Queenie, a deaf woman living in a small town in Ireland, memories of a summer night twenty years ago.

The house in which her rooms were was so familiar that she went upstairs without a pause in the dark. Crossing her sitting-room she smelled oil from the cooker behind the screen: she went through an arch to the cubicle where she slept. She was happy. Inside her sphere of silence that not a word clouded, the spectacle of the evening at Bellevue reigned. Contemplative, wishless, almost without an 'I', she unhooked her muslin dress at the wrists and waist, stepped from the dress and began to take down her hair. Still in the dark, with a dreaming sureness of habit, she dropped hairpins into the heart-shaped tray.

This was the night she knew she would find again. It had stayed living under a film of time. On just such a summer night, once only, she had walked with a lover in the demesne. His hand, like Robinson's, had been on her elbow, but she had guided him, not he her, because she had better eyes in the dark. They had gone down walks already deadened with moss, under the weight of July trees; they had felt the then fresh aghast ruin totter above them; there was a moonless sky. Beside the lake they sat down, and while her hand brushed the ferns in the cracks of the stone seat emanations of kindness passed from him to her. The subtle deaf girl had made the transposition of this nothing or everything into an everything – the delicate deaf girl that the man could not speak to and was afraid to touch. She who, then so deeply contented, kept in her senses each frond and breath of that night, never saw him again and had soon forgotten his face. That had been twenty years ago, till tonight, when it was now. Tonight it was Robinson who, guided by Queenie down leaf tunnels, took the place on the stone seat by the lake.

The rusted gates of the castle were at the end of the square. Queenie, in her bed facing the window, lay with her face turned sideways, smiling, one hand lightly against her cheek.

From 'Summer Night', in *The Collected Stories of Elizabeth Bowen*

Having escaped from the narrator, who had been her lover, Lolita [Dolly] marries Dick. Too poor to travel to Alaska, where Dick has been offered work, Lolita applies to her former lover for financial help. This leads to his visit to Lolita's new home, where he meets Dick, who believes him to be Lolita's father, and Bill, a neighbour.

'Dick's down there,' she said pointing with an invisible tennis racket, inviting my gaze to travel from the drab parlour-bedroom where we stood, right across the kitchen, and through the back-doorway where in a rather primitive vista, a dark-haired young stranger in overalls, instantaneously reprieved, was perched with his back to me on a ladder fixing something near or upon the shack of his neighbour, a plumper fellow with only one arm, who stood looking up.

This pattern, she explained from afar, apologetically ('Men will be men'); should she call him in?

No . . .

At this point, there came brisk homey sounds from the kitchen into which Dick and Bill had lumbered in quest of beer. Through the doorway they noticed the visitor, and Dick entered the parlour.

'Dick, this is my Dad!' cried Dolly in a resounding violent voice that struck me as totally strange, and new, and cheerful, and old, and sad, because the young fellow, veteran of a remote war was hard of hearing . . .

They were under the impression I had come to stay, and Dick with a great wrinkling of brows that denoted difficult thought, suggested Dolly and he might sleep in the kitchen on a spare mattress. I waved a light hand and told Dolly who transmitted it by means of a special shout to Dick that I had merely dropped in on my way to Readsburg where I was to be entertained by some friends and admirers. It was then noticed that one of the few thumbs remaining to Bill was bleeding (not such a wonderworker after all). How womanish and somehow never seen that way before was the shadowy division between her pale breasts when she bent down over the man's hand! She took him for repairs to the kitchen. For a few minutes, three or four little eternities which positively welled with artificial warmth, Dick and I remained alone. He sat on a hard chair rubbing his forelimbs and frowning . . .

Good. If he was silent I could be silent, too. Indeed, I could very well do with a little rest in this subdued, frightened-to-death rocking chair . . . But presently I became sorry for poor Dick whom, in some hypnotoid way, I was horribly preventing from making the only remark he could think up ('She's a swell kid . . .').

'And so,' I said, 'you are going to Canada?'

In the kitchen, Dolly was laughing at something Bill had said or done.

'And so,' I shouted, 'you are going to Canada? Not Canada' – I re-shouted – 'I mean Alaska, of course.'

He nursed his glass and, nodding sagely, replied: 'Well, he cut it on a jagger, I guess. Lost his right arm in Italy.'

Lonely mauve almond trees in bloom. A blown-off surrealistic arm hanging up there in the pointillistic mauve. A flowergirl tattoo on the hand. Dolly and band-aided Bill reappeared. It occurred to me that her ambiguous, brown and pale beauty excited the cripple. Dick, with a grin of relief stood up. He guessed Bill and he would be going back to fix those wires. He guessed he would be seeing me before I left. Why do these people guess so much and shave so little, and are so disdainful of hearing aids?

From *Lolita*

Jo, whose hearing has been miraculously restored by an operation, receives advice from the surgeon who carried it out, as she prepares to go home. The authenticity of this novel is explained by the fact that Lady Packer's son was an ear surgeon and that she took a great interest in his operations and the experiences of his patients.

. . . James warned me that for a while everything would sound strange and often frightening.

'Sounds may echo in your head like cries in an empty house. That will pass as things settle down. Many noises you've forgotten may scare you. You'll soon get used to them again. The world is a very noisy place, Jo. You're back in it.'

'That's what I want. To be back in it!' In the tide of life, buffeted perhaps, but no longer isolated.

'I suggest putting a light sound-resistant plug in your ear for a day or two, so you can adjust gradually.'

'No! I'll take it as it is and really live again.'

Their voices did indeed echo as if in a cave.

Outside when Rob drove me home, I had to control sheer terror.

The noises seemed deafening – or so anybody else would say. To me the word 'deafening' has a different meaning. The traffic and the stormy weather! They assaulted the newly opened door of my ear and rushed at that sensitive threshold from all directions as if to burst into my head and create havoc there. It was mad and Wagnerian – a sort of Götterdämmerung of sound. The rain and the wind thundered out of the heavens like the galloping Valkyries. Cars, vans, and motorbikes whooshed, roared, growled, whined, hooted and snarled in a mechanical cacophony I had long forgotten. No wonder wheels were the killers of to-day. Listen to them! Each noise was a separate threat to which the hard-of-hearing are oblivious. Often, on foot, I had risked my life inadvertently, and horns had blared, teeth gnashed and fists shaken in fury at the stupidity of the 'jay-walker' impeding the path of speed and the power of the man at the wheel.

My heart thumped as I realised that soon I must be prepared to plunge into all this turmoil and drive my car again, not just with hands, feet and eyes, but with ears alert to every warning . . .

It was the same in the quiet flat.

Mummy and Gert met us at the door. My little son's footsteps, scampering across the polished floor of the hall, were like the hooves of a wild pony, and his cry of welcome was as penetrating as a steam whistle when he flung himself upon me.

'Mom! Mom! Can you hear?'

I knelt on the doormat, remembering even then, James Sherrard's advice not to make hasty movements with my head. Gert was in my arms and I was hugging him.

'I can hear, darling. You need never shout at me again!'

From *Boomerang*

Maurice, Lady Eliot's son by her first marriage, is about to marry Diana. Godfrey, a friend, breaks the news to Maurice's mother and his stepfather that she is 'handicapped'.

'She has a limp. It looks like the kind of limp that polio leaves them with, but I believe she's always had it.'

'Is it very bad?'

'One is aware of it. Perhaps it's more distressing to others than to herself. I think, taken alone, no, it is not very bad.'

'Taken alone? You mean there's something else?'

'She is also partially deaf,' said Godfrey, 'I think that is congenital too, and she has never had normal hearing. Of course, that made her backward as a child. But mentally she has caught up. I mustn't give you the impression that she is brilliant. There is nothing wrong with her there, though. What is more serious is that being deaf has kept her out of things. She is very uncertain of herself, I doubt whether she has ever made friends. And that is why Maurice has changed everything for her.'

'Is that what he means,' said Margaret, voice tight, 'when he says she's handicapped?'

'That is what he means.' . . .

Three weeks later, I was able to see Maurice's wife for myself. He brought her to tea one afternoon, and trying to settle her down and to smooth away her shyness (and our own), Margaret and I complained heartily of the misty weather, and made a parade of drawing the curtains and shutting the evening out.

'Oh never mind,' said Maurice, entirely serene. 'It'll be worse where we live, won't it, darling?'

His wife didn't reply, but she understood, and gave a dependent trusting smile . . .

She hadn't a feature which one noticed much, but she wasn't either in the English or the American sense, homely. Often she wore the expression, at the same time puzzled, obstinate, and protesting that one saw in the chronically deaf. How deaf she was, I couldn't tell. Maurice spoke to her with the words slowed down, deliberately using the muscles of his lips, and she seemed to follow him easily. Sometimes he had to interpret for Margaret and me . . .

We should have had to quarry for conversation if it hadn't been for Maurice, but he took charge, like an adoring young husband acting as impresario. Each time he spoke to her, she smiled as though he had once more called her into existence . . .

I did manage to have one exchange with her, but it couldn't have been called specially illuminating. I had been casting round, heavy-footed, for gossip about the Manchester district. I happened to mention the United football team. Her eyes suddenly brightened and became sharp, not puzzled: she had heard me, she gave a sky-blue recognising glance. Yes, she liked football. She supported the United. There wasn't a team like them anywhere. She used to go to their matches – 'until I met him'. It was the first time she had referred to Maurice without directly speaking to him, and they were both laughing. 'I'm not much good to you about that, am I?' said Maurice, who had no more interest in competitive games than in competing at anything himself.

From *Last Things*

144

Miss Dredger is upset by the behaviour of Mr Pye, her new lodger.

The insufferable nerve of the little man had caught her unawares, but that sort of thing must end immediately. Here, on her own ground, she would stand no nonsense.

She marched to the kitchen where Ka-Ka, a very old woman, was stirring up the wrong ingredients in the wrong bowl at the wrong time. Old Ka-Ka's idea of a *vol-au-vent* was entirely her own. She was blind in one eye, completely deaf, and had a cleft palate.

This was very sad, but Miss Dredger could not be sympathetic all the time. The milk of human kindness has a way of turning when things go wrong, and Miss Dredger plucked the pastry-board from the old woman and threw the dreadful contents out of the window.

Immediately, a black-backed gull landed beside the jetsam, straddled its way around it, squinting at the mess from every direction, and then, in spite of its hunger and the jaded condition of its palate, flapped away peevishly.

Miss Dredger raised her hands to the level of Ka-Ka's one remaining eye and spelt out in deaf-and-dumb language the uncompromising message, which after several attempts was interpreted eventually as 'Go home'.

She would have to prepare another kind of lunch altogether and, if it was late, Mr Pye could bally well wait for it.

From *Mr Pye*

Singer's friend Antonapoulos, deaf without speech like Singer himself, has become mentally deranged and is committed to an asylum in a distant town.

The weeks that followed did not seem real at all. All day Singer worked over his bench in the back of the jewelry store, and then at night he returned to the house alone. More than anything he wanted to sleep. As soon as he came home from work he would lie on his cot and try to doze awhile. Dreams came to him when he lay there half-asleep. And in all of them Antonapoulos was there. His hands would jerk nervously, for in his dreams he was talking to his friend and Antonapoulos was watching him.

Singer tried to think of the time before he had ever known his friend. He tried to recount to himself certain things that had happened when he was young. But none of these things he tried to remember seemed real.

There was one particular fact he remembered, but it was not at all important to him. Singer recalled that, although he had been deaf since he was an infant, he had not always been a real mute. He was left an orphan very young and placed in an institution for the deaf. He had learned to talk with his hands and read. Before he was nine years old he could talk with one hand in the American way – and also could employ both of his hands after the method of Europeans. He had learned to follow the movements of people's lips and to understand what they said. Then finally he had been taught to speak.

At the school he was thought very intelligent. He learned the lessons before the rest of the pupils. But he could never become used to speaking with his lips. It was not natural to him, and his tongue felt like a whale in his mouth. From the blank expression on people's faces to whom he talked in this way he felt that his voice must be like the sound of some animal or that there was something disgusting in his speech. It was painful for him to try to talk with his mouth, but his hands were always ready to shape the words he wished to say. When he was twenty-two he had come South to this town from Chicago and he met Antonapoulos immediately. Since that time he had never spoken with his mouth again, because with his friend there was no need for this.

Nothing seemed real except the ten years with Antonapoulos. In his half-dream he saw his friend very vividly, and when he awakened a great aching loneliness would be in him. Occasionally he would pack up a box for Antonapoulos, but he never received any reply. And so the months passed in this empty, dreaming way.

On one of his visits to the asylum Singer learns that his friend has died.

The afternoon was almost ended when a strange thing happened to Singer. He had been walking slowly and irregularly along the curb of the street. The sky was overcast and the air humid. Singer did not raise his head, but as he passed the town pool room he caught a sidewise glance of something that disturbed him. He passed the pool room and then stopped in the middle of the street. Listlessly he retraced his steps and stood before the open door of the place. There were three mutes inside and they were talking with their hands together. All three of them were coatless. They wore bowler hats and bright ties. Each of them held a glass of beer in his left hand. There was a certain brotherly resemblance between them.

Singer went inside. For a moment he had trouble taking his hand from his pocket. Then clumsily he formed a word of greeting. He was clapped on the shoulder. A cold drink was ordered. They surrounded him and the fingers of their hands shot out like pistons as they questioned him.

He told his own name and the name of the town where he lived. After that he could think of nothing else to tell about himself. He asked if they knew Spiros Antonapoulos. They did not know him. Singer stood with his hands dangling loose. His head was still inclined to one side and his glance was oblique. He was so listless and cold that the three mutes in the bowler hats looked at him queerly. After a while they left him out of their conversation. And when they had paid for the rounds of beers and were ready to depart they did not suggest that he join them.

Although Singer had been adrift on the streets for half a day he almost missed his train. It was not clear to him how this happened or how he had spent the hours before. He reached the station two minutes before the train pulled out, and barely had time to drag his luggage aboard and find a seat. The car he chose was almost empty. ... At midnight he drew the window-shade and lay down on the seat. He was curled in a ball, his coat pulled over his face and head. In this position he lay in a stupor of half-sleep for about twelve hours. The conductor had to shake him when they arrived.

Singer left his luggage in the middle of the station floor. Then he walked to the shop. He greeted the jeweler for whom he worked with a listless turn of his hand. When he went out again there was something heavy in his pocket. For a while he rambled with bent head along the streets. But the unrefracted brilliance of the sun, the humid heat, oppressed him. He returned to his room with swollen eyes and an aching head. After resting he drank a glass of iced coffee and smoked a cigarette. Then when he had washed the ash tray and the glass he brought out a pistol from his pocket and put a bullet in his chest.

From *The Heart Is a Lonely Hunter*

Arcas, a Cretan resistance fighter, escaped with his life, but lost his hearing, when the Germans blew up his hide-out. After the war, he joins a gang of grave robbers out of a sense of bitterness and frustration.

found myself almost at peace, perhaps because there was nothing p here to hear which I couldn't imagine: the sound of the spring, ome birds, a rustle of leaves in the afternoon breeze from time to me, and a child chattering to himself as he played; sometimes he poke to me, but a smile and a nod were more than he expected in nswer and his own smile split his round face with almond vhiteness.

didn't even know what I was myself conveying when I spoke. If ou can't hear what you say, you cannot be absolutely certain that ou've said it and when you get an unexpected reaction from omeone you wonder if your speech is getting out of your control: nd in any case, you cannot, of course, be sure of the tone you have .sed.

could think only with great self-pity that it was very hard to be a eaf man, because you must always appear slow and clumsy and omething of a coward since it took so long to understand other ·eople. I realised suddenly that probably I was truly a coward ompared with other men, because all alarm, emergency and fright re enhanced and made much worse if you are a sense short: a urious man whom you can only see, without hearing what he is ellowing at you, is terrifying because only partly understood.

'anni was one of those who never learnt that nothing can make a eaf man hear: he always poured out a great many words, with

violent but not very evocative gestures: also, he shook his he
sometimes for 'yes' and sometimes for 'no', nodding it for '»
only. This is a difficulty – at least for a deaf man – in Greece, wh«
some of us are more Eastern than we care to admit. When you get
Istanbul, they say, a nod is invariably 'no' and a headshake 'yes»
said, knowing he would not, having in the five years since he l
school at twelve almost forgotten how, 'You must write for me.' I
shook his head and then nodded violently and began a combir
tion of acting, miming and making signs . . . with extraordin;
energy and grace and a humour and imagination I had not thoug
he possessed. He was a noted performer in the bazoukia an«
suppose once he had made up his mind to make me understar
the whole thing seemed to him a kind of interpretative dance. I :
on the little wall, laughing and occasionally applauding, telling h
what I had understood, questioning and laughing again as
laughed back in triumph . . . It must have taken ten minutes befc
I thought I had found out all that was going on, or, at least, tł
Yanni knew was going on.

The only obstacle [to breaking away from the gang] was tha
couldn't hear. I was used enough to silence, which is, in its w;
often truly golden, even when you have nothing else. The fear I
in the sight of strangers' lips moving, the knowledge that they w«
talking together about you, probably against you and often to y«
shouting at you, even though they could hear you saying tł
nothing could make you hear. Stone deaf. But no one tries to talk
stones. It was hard to face the reluctant taking of the pad of pa;
and pencil, the diffident, unskilled writing of a word or two w;
hesitations over spelling and the result which, as often as n
would be pointless questions written instead of the informati
asked for. You would think people were themselves deaf when
who was, tried to communicate with them.
  'Greek?'
  'Yes, I'm Greek, but I'm deaf, stone deaf.'
  'French?'
  Surely I still speak clearly?
  'I'm Greek, I'm stone deaf, however.'
  They talk to each other. One of them writes again: 'Can't hea

'No. I'm deaf. An accident. Can you tell me when the boat leaves
or Piraeus?'

Could I face it?

From *The Cretan*

Elizabeth Ayrton writes in a letter to the editor:

wrote *The Cretan* in the sixties, mainly because I wanted to write
bout Cretan archaeology, in which I have retained a passionate
nterest ever since I first went to Crete in 1956. As I conceived the
tory I needed a hero-figure with some disability. For various
easons I was interested in the effect of a physical disaster imposed
·y an accident of peace or war on a young man who had previously
hought of himself as mentally and physically as good as, or better
han, his peer group (and, indeed, others).

I didn't want to write about a purely physical disaster, such as
he loss of a limb; I couldn't write about blindness, nor would the
tory have been possible. When I began to think about deafness, I
·new that that was what had happened to my central character.

I talked to various medical friends and read a good deal about
leafness and became very much interested in what this would be
·ke in a poor, rather isolated community, where first-class medical,
urgical and psychological treatment were not immediately and
·bviously available. It seemed to me that if you were already very
ngry and very secret (as most Cretans were after the German
nvasion of the island) deafness, suddenly imposed, would drive
he victim so far into himself that he would feel an even greater
lespair than the deaf almost always feel. In the case of my
·rotagonist his helpless rage was so great that he refused even to
ry to get help in lip-reading or for the actual condition.

I am getting rather deaf myself in my seventies, but this is a
;radual, quite gentle, mildly irritating process. I am part of a large
amily all living together here most of the time and, though I think I
ay 'What'?' more than anyone else does, no one seems to mind.
Jothing could be more different from this than sudden complete
leafness imposed by outside forces early in life.

Portrait of a deaf watchmaker.

The deaf watchmaker, Simon Datnow, was employed by Kate father in his jeweller's shop. I've got a lot of time for Simon, M Shand would say consideredly, with a 'mind you', a sage reserv tion in her voice. That was because, on the whole, she did not ca for relatives, and this man was, in fact, one of the procession Lithuanian and Russian relatives whom Marcus Shand h 'brought out' to South Africa, before Kate was born, in the ear twenties, and whom, ever after, he regarded with a surly indiffe ence quite out of character with his gentle nature – a churlishne created by the conflict in him between family feeling for them, an a resentment against them for being the kind of people he wou not have expected his wife to like . . .

Simon Datnow was not actually a blood relation of Marc Shand, but merely the brother of one of Mr Shand's siste husbands. The husband was dead and Simon had 'come out' wi his sister-in-law as a kind of substitute protector. Perhaps it w because there was no blood-tie to rein his resentment with gu that, if Mrs Shand liked Simon most, Mr Shand liked him least the immigrant relations. It seemed to annoy Marcus Shand th after the first year, the deaf watchmaker really owed him nothin had, unlike the others, nothing in particular for which to grateful to him. Simon Datnow had paid back the passage mon which Mr Shand had advanced, and he was a skilled watchmak whose equal Mr Shand could not have hoped to find in Sou Africa. Kate always remembered the watchmaker as she used to s him from the door, whenever she entered her father's shop, sitti in his little three-sided glass cage with the inscription, in gold le WATCH REPAIR DEPARTMENT, showing like a banner across his be head. As Kate grew up, the gold leaf began to peel, and behind t faint loop of the first P, you could see his left ear more and mo clearly. In that ear, from time to time, a new hearing-aid, fles coloured, black or pearly, would appear, but usually, when he w

vorking, he did not wear one. He would put it on only when you
ipproached to speak to him, and in the moment before you did
›peak, the moment when the device dropped into contact with his
ar, you would see him wince as the roar of the world, from which
ie had been sealed off like a man dropped in a diving-bell to the
loor of the ocean, burst in upon him . . .

Summer and winter, most days he looked up only when Marcus
Shand came stumping over to shove at him a watch for diagnosis,
›ellowing 'Loses twenty-five minutes in twenty-four hours' or
Oiling and cleaning. See if it's in working order.' 'What?' the deaf
nan would say in his sibilant, half-audible voice, frowning
acantly and fumbling for his 'machine' – as he always called his
iearing-aid – while he held back from the force of his employer in
iervous distaste. Shand would shout in impatient repetition, so
hat half of what he said would not be heard by the watchmaker,
ind the other half would thunder in upon him as his aid was
 witched on. The force of this half-sentence would strike the
vatchmaker like a blow, so that for a moment he was bewildered
ind unable to understand anything. Then Shand would become
nore impatient than ever, and shout twice as loud. Because of this
:ommunication at cross purposes, Marcus Shand tended to phrase
iverything he had to say to his watchmaker as shortly as possible,
ind to dispense with all graces of politeness, and so almost all that
ame to Simon Datnow of the outside world for eight hours a day
vas an assault of surly questions and demands.

Because his watchmaker and relation by marriage was sensitive
o the tick of a watch but not an undertone of the human voice,
Marcus Shand got into the habit of abusing Simon Datnow in
numbled asides, before his very face. It was a great comfort to
Shand to be able to abuse someone with impunity. Yet although it
vas true that he was able to say abusive things without being
ieard, it was, of course, not possible for these not to show on his
ace while he said them, and so it was that Simon Datnow felt the
evilement more cuttingly than if it had come to him in words, and
ı wall of thick, inarticulate hostility, far more impenetrable than
hat of deafness, came to exist between the two men . . .

One day, a week before Christmas in the year when Kate was
iine years old, she was hanging about her father's shop . . . On this
›articular day, Simon Datnow was so busy that the face of the little

girl, who had wandered over to watch him through the glass, d
not penetrate his concentration. She watched him a minute or tw
nevertheless. He fitted a tiny spring into the intricacy of a watch
belly; over it went a wheel; into some pin-sized holes, three chip
of ruby. Then he put out his long tweezers, to peck from i
spirit-bath something that proved not to be there; he felt abo
with the tweezers, looked in another dish; at last, lifted h
eyebrow so that the jeweller's loop in his left eye-socket fell o
into his hand. He stood up from his stool and looked carefully ar
methodically under every glass bell, in every dish. He rummage
systematically through the cardboard box-lid where he kept th
filings, little twirls of yellow and silver metal like punctuatic
marks, from the watchstraps, the necklaces, the bracelets. I
paused a moment, as if deliberating where he should look nex
And then, the light of a solution, a calm relief relaxed his fac
Slowly, he stood back, creaking his stool away behind him over th
cement floor. Then he grasped his work table firmly, palms t
under its top, and brought it over, crashing and slithering all i
conglomeration of contents on top of himself.

He stood there with his hands hanging at his sides, amid th
wreckage. His eyes glittered and his mouth clenched, so that th
skin, in which the growing beard showed like fine blue shot, w
white above and below his stiffened lips. He was breathing
loudly that it could be heard right across the sudden silence of th
shop full of people.

Before the shock of that silence broke, Kate ran. Her runnir
broke the silence; she heard, as she pulled the heavy back door
the shop closed behind her, babble and movement spill out . .

When she went back into the shop again, there was a cheerf
delegation of a mine, in the part of the shop known as the jewelle
department, choosing a canteen of cutlery for presentation to
retiring official. Behind the WATCH REPAIR DEPARTMENT, th
watchmaker was putting the last of his tiny containers back at th
angle at which it had always stood; only the glass bells we
missing, and they must have been swept away by Albert, th
African cleaner. The face of the watchmaker, behind the gold-le
letters, was pale and calm.

Presently, he looked up and beckoned to her across the sho
and, hesitantly, she went to him. He gave her one of the thre

:ornered buns filled with poppyseed which he had brought for his ea, and he knew she loved. Holding it between finger and thumb, ;he took the bun to the back room and hid it in a corner, for the nice.

From 'Charmed Lives', in *Six Feet of the Country*

> The most striking fact about these deaf men and women is that they were *not* handicapped, because no one perceived their deafness as a handicap. As one woman said to me, 'You know, we didn't think anything special about them. They were just like anyone else.'*
>
> Nora Ellen Groce

* This comment concludes the book of this anthropologist's investigation of the incidence of hereditary deafness on Martha's Vineyard, Massachusetts. On the island, from the seventeenth to the early twentieth century, there existed amongst the population an exceptionally high rate of profoundly deaf people. 'The residents compensated for this condition by inventing or borrowing an efficient sign language, which was used by almost everyone, hearing and deaf alike' (from *Everyone Here Spoke Sign Language*, 1985).

*The canonisation of Philip of Evesham, a seventeenth-century
monk, is the subject of Prudence Andrew's historical novel. His
brother's testimony forms part of the evidence for consideration by
the Church.*

It was a good time afore the day come for Philip to start talking. I'
watch him often, lying tight bound in his swaddling with a fis'
under his chin, never crying. He got a queer face for a baba, long
and white under his red hair, with black eyebrows and black eyes
and blue veins in his forehead and a valley between his nose and
his lip . . . I got to taking him with me in a basket when I was
ploughing, hanging him in a tree so as he could watch me . . .

. . . He was deaf. Deaf and dumb. There was something stopping
his ears and a chain on his tongue and he never uttered nor heard
nothing.

Soon as it was certain, my Dad told the priest and of course it got
round to Brother Roger at the priory and he said it must be devils
There was some believed him at first and said my Mum and Dad
must have sinned terrible to have a child possessed by the devil.
Brother Roger was all for beating the devil out of him. 'He'll speak
soon enough when he feels the lash on his back,' he said, but the
priest wouldn't let him.

He was Philip's friend from the start, that priest. Father Francis
he was, a Norman man but spoke English beautiful and that good
there was no one dared lay hands on Philip, not once he'd given
out there wasn't no devil in the boy. Brother Roger kept it up long
enough, as you'll be hearing, but then he'd have seen a devil in
paradise, I do believe.

He was a lovely child. There wasn't no one outside the priory but
come to love him. My dad grizzled on times when he shouted at
him and nothing happened but once you'd got him to see what was
needful he was quick enough. He got a way of flinging his arms
and legs about, too, to show what he wanted to say . . .

Brother Roger said Philip got a devil in him but I reckoned it was

156

all my eye and told him so straight. What if he couldn't talk? There's others been the same surely and gone to Heaven. Proper little angel he was. He seemed to listen on times, for all he couldn't hear. You'd find him with the pigs in the woods or scraping dung in the road and he'd be listening, like he heard someone talking to him. 'It's angels,' said my Mum. He couldn't stand blood, nor any pain nor suffering, and when there was a whipping or a pair of ears cropped or a branding Mum used to take him in the house and set him to scraping the hen perches.

And devout! I never know a nipper take to church like he done. I never give it much thought at the time, being courting. But come to think of it, it was queer he should take to church and that like he did. I mean, he couldn't know, could he? About the Holy Sacraments and the Mass and Confession and the rest of it? He couldn't hear when the priest told the other boys about it and how they were eating God's body when they swallowed the wafer, and how they'd got to confess their sins regular in case they died sudden without a priest near and went to Hell. Not that I ever known him sin, not bad. Father Francis used to absolve him along of the others just in case. I don't reckon he had any sins.

But Brother Roger said he had. He even had a go at stopping Philip's first Communion. What a do that was! I never seen Father Francis so mad. He got them all up at the altar rail, the girls with them white things over their heads and the boys with their hair cut, and he got to the bit where he says *Est enim corpus*, or something like, when in bust Brother Roger waving his arms and tripping over people's feet. He grabbed hold of Philip and made to lug him away and Philip went white as snow and clung to the rail like he was drowning. Cried too but silent like he always did, with his mouth open and nothing coming out of it and the tears dripping on to his chest.

'Devils! Devils!' yelled Brother Roger, tugging Philip's coat. 'Do you want devils to eat God's body?'

Up came my Dad then and clouted Brother Roger, so he let go of Philip and fell down on the pavement. I got my arms round my Dad to stop him bashing Brother Roger again and my Mum screamed and Philip fainted. I'll not forget seeing him hanging over the rail like he'd been broken on a wheel, with his arms dangling.

Father Francis was still stood there with God in his hands. He said to Brother Roger: 'How dare you disturb the peace of God's house? There are no devils in Philip Ganter and he shall partake of God's body with the rest. Out of here now before I bloody your nose.'

Brother Roger slunk away like a rat and soon as he had gone Philip come to and the Mass went on and they had their Communion in peace.

From *Ordeal by Silence*

Who is so deafe, or so blynde, as is hee,
that wilfully will nother here nor see?

From John Heywood's
Collection of English Proverbs

None so deaf as those who will not hear.

Modern version of the same proverb

'The Deaf Man', a master criminal, passes himself off as a detective.

The rain lashed the windows of the bar on Jefferson Avenue, some three and a half miles southwest of the station house. The tall blond man with the hearing aid in his right ear had just told Naomi he was a cop. A police *detective*, no less. She didn't know the police department was hiring deaf people nowadays. Anti-discrimination laws, she supposed. They allowed you to hire *anybody*. Next you'd have detectives who were midgets. Not that a hearing aid necessarily meant you were deaf. Not stone *cold* deaf anyway. Still she guessed any degree of hearing loss could be considered an infirmity, and she was far too polite to ask him how a man wearing a hearing aid had passed the physical examinations she supposed the police department required. Some people were sensitive about such things.

He was good-looking.

For a cop.

From *Eight Black Horses*

Zipser, research graduate of Porterhouse College, calls on the college chaplain for advice about his uncontrollable sexual longing for Mrs Biggs, his bedder.

'Ah my boy,' the Chaplain boomed as Zipser negotiated the bric-a-brac that filled the Chaplain's sitting room. 'So good of you to come. Do make yourself comfortable.' . . .

The Chaplain sat back in his chair and filled his pipe from a tobacco jar with the Porterhouse crest on it.

'Do help yourself, my dear boy,' said the Chaplain, pushing the jar towards him.

'I don't smoke.'

The Chaplain shook his head sadly. 'Everyone should smoke a pipe,' he said. 'Calms the nerves. Puts things in perspective. Couldn't do without mine.' He leant back, puffing vigorously. Zipser stared at him through a haze of smoke.

'Now then where were we?' he asked. Zipser tried to think.

'Ah yes, your little problem, that's right,' said the Chaplain finally. 'I knew there was something.'

Zipser stared into the fire resentfully.

'The Senior Tutor said something about it. I didn't gather very much but then I seldom do. Deafness, you know.'

Zipser nodded sympathetically.

'The affliction of the elderly. That and rheumatism. It's the damp, you know. Comes up from the river. Very unhealthy living so close to the Fens.' His pipe percolated gently. In the comparative silence Zipser tried to think what to say. The Chaplain's age and his evident physical disabilities made it difficult for Zipser to conceive that he could begin to understand the problem of Mrs Biggs.

'I really think there's been a misunderstanding,' he began hesitantly and stopped. It was evident from the look on the Chaplain's face that there was no understanding at all.

'You'll have to speak up,' the Chaplain boomed. 'I'm really quite deaf.'

'I can see that,' Zipser said. The Chaplain beamed at him.

'Don't hesitate to tell me,' he said. 'Nothing you say can shock me.'

'I'm not surprised,' Zipser said.

The Chaplain's smile remained insistently benevolent. 'I know what we'll do,' he said, hopping to his feet and reaching behind his chair. 'It's something I use for confession sometimes.' He emerged holding a loudhailer and handed it to Zipser. 'Press the trigger when you're going to speak.'

Zipser held the thing up to his mouth and stared at the Chaplain over the rim. 'I really don't think this is going to help,' he said finally. His words reverberated through the room and set the teapot rattling on the brass table.

'Of course it is,' shouted the Chaplain, 'I can hear perfectly.'

'I didn't mean that,' Zipser said desperately. The fronds of the castor-oil plant quivered ponderously. 'I meant I don't think it's going to help to talk about . . .' He left the dilemma of Mrs Biggs unspoken.

The Chaplain smiled in absolution and puffed his pipe vigorously. 'Many of the young men who come to see me,' he said, invisible in a cloud of smoke, 'suffer from feelings of guilt about masturbation.'

Zipser stared frantically at the smokescreen. 'Masturbation? Who said anything about masturbation?' he bawled into the loudhailer. It was apparent someone had. His words, hideously amplified, billowed forth from the room and across the Court outside. Several undergraduates by the fountain turned and stared up at the Chaplain's windows. Deafened by his own vociferousness Zipser sat sweating with embarrassment.

'I understood from the Senior Tutor that you wanted to see me about a sexual problem,' the Chaplain shouted.

Zipser lowered the loudhailer. The thing clearly had disadvantages. 'I can assure you I don't masturbate,' he said.

The Chaplain looked at him incomprehendingly. 'You press the trigger when you want to speak,' he explained. Zipser nodded dumbly.

The knowledge that to communicate with the Chaplain at all he had to announce his feelings for Mrs Biggs to the world at large presented him with a terrible dilemma made no less intolerable by the Chaplain's shouted replies.

'It often helps to get these things into the open,' the Chaplain assured him. Zipser had his doubts about that. Admissions of the sort he had to make broadcast through a loudhailer were not likely to be of any help at all. He might just as well go and propose to the wretched woman straightaway and be done with it. He sat with lowered head while the Chaplain boomed on.

'Don't forget that anything you tell me will be heard in the strictest confidence,' he shouted. 'You need have no fears that it will go any further.'

'Oh sure,' Zipser muttered. Outside in the Quad a small crowd of undergraduates had gathered by the fountain to listen.

Half an hour later Zipser left the room, his demoralisation quite complete.

From *Porterhouse Blue*

Colin Dexter, the crime novelist, has been profoundly deaf since his mid-twenties. In this novel, set in Oxford where he works as a university administrator, he has created a deaf murder victim. Here, Chief Inspector Morse pays a visit to the lip-reading class which Quinn, the dead man, had attended.

As Morse looked at the Thursday-evening class with their hearing aids, private or NHS, plugged into their ears, he reminded himself that during the previous weeks of the term Quinn had sat there amongst his fellow-students, sharing the mysteries and the silent manifestations. There were eight of them, sitting in a single row in front of their teacher, and at the back of the room Morse felt that he was watching a TV screen with the sound turned off. The teacher was talking, for her lips moved and she made the natural gestures of speech. But no sound. When Morse had managed to rid himself of the suspicion that *he* had been suddenly struck deaf, he watched the teacher's lips more closely, and tried as hard as he could to read the words. Occasionally one or other of the class would raise a hand and voice a silent question, and then the teacher would write up a word on the blackboard. Frequently, it appeared, the difficult words – the words that the class were puzzled by – began with 'p', or 'b', or 'm'; and to a lesser extent with 't', 'd', or 'n'. Lip-reading was clearly a most sophisticated skill.

At the end of the class, Morse thanked the teacher for allowing him to observe, and spoke to her about Quinn. Here, too, he had been the star pupil, it seemed, and all the class had been deeply upset at the news of his death. Yes, he really had been very deaf indeed – but one wouldn't have guessed; unless, that is, one had experience of these things.

A bell sounded throughout the building. It was 9 p.m. and time for everyone to leave the premises.

'Would he have been able to hear that?' asked Morse.

But the teacher had temporarily turned away to mark the register. The bell was still ringing. 'Would Quinn have been able to hear that?' repeated Morse.

But she still didn't hear him, and, belatedly, Morse guessed the truth. When finally she looked up again, he repeated his question once more.

'Could Quinn hear the bell?'

'Could Quinn hear them all, did you say? I'm sorry, I didn't quite catch—'

'H-ear th-e b-e-ll,' mouthed Morse, with ridiculous exaggeration.

'Oh, the *bell*. Is it ringing? I'm afraid that none of us could ever hear that.'

From *The Silent World of Nicholas Quinn*

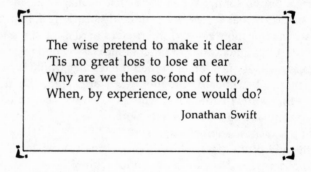

The wise pretend to make it clear
'Tis no great loss to lose an ear
Why are we then so fond of two,
When, by experience, one would do?

Jonathan Swift

JOANNE GREENBERG 1932–

*Abel Ryder, the principal character in Joanne Greenberg's novel,
thinks back to his first day at school in rural America. Born deaf and
son of a deaf father and hearing mother, the day has a special
significance for him.*

His mother had taken his clothes and set them out by the stove.
She motioned him to get dressed. Church clothes, but it isn't
church-day. He began to show his mother it was a wood-day,
sawing back and forth, the tree-fall. She laughed, but didn't look
happy. She made her mouth into something he did not know, a
mouth 'Uuuuuu'. Then Breakfast. Afterwards she kissed him,
making with her hand: 'Outside'. And there was the wagon and
his father sitting up on it, waiting and making 'Uuuuuu' with his
mouth. Abel also tried 'Uuuuuu', and they looked at one another
until his mother looked away. His mother was a Hearing. He only
knew it later. Then he looked down at himself in his nice clothes.
But Uuuuuu is not a church-day.

Not church? They rode away from town, a way only gone when
they went to visit the molasses-eating people. His mother was
always trying to show or tell him something, but he could never
find it. His mother's mouth was always trying to make him do and
feel and the things were always mysteries that made him tired and
angry. His father did not show with his mouth.

Children were on the road. His father stopped the cart and
motioned them: Come up. They did and again and again until
there were many. Then Abel had an idea. He was going where they
were going. He got frightened. He did not want to keep moving
towards that place. They went farther than he ever was, far past the
house of the molasses-eating people. They turned in then and
stopped at a building with a top made of stone.

A woman came out and there were children running and playing
all around. Only children. There was a church bell hung on a
slaughtering-frame-thing on the far side. The woman went over
and pulled a rope and the bell-feeling went through Abel so that

his teeth began to pull themselves inside his head and his face bones shook weak under his skin. The riding children opened their mouths and fell off the cart and everywhere they ran and ran, into the building.

His father leaned down and took up an egg box and showed it to him, opened it so that he could see the food inside and gave it to him. Then his father pushed him towards the edge of the seat and nodded and looked towards the building where all the children were swallowed. He made 'Uuuuuu', and Abel knew that this was Uuuuuu. He got down, his face cold and his body feeling stiff and tired. He held the egg box tightly and went to the door. When he was almost there, he turned and looked back. The cart was pulled around and was moving away from him down the road.

Inside was large, and so much with things that for a long time he only stared. There was a sour-yellow smell of damp, cold, old, and bad-boy. The bad-boy reminded him that he needed to go to the backhouse. His stomach hurt with that. But the room held him, and only when he felt the first drops beginning did he turn and run. A girl was coming out of it and he almost ran into her at the door. She said something too fast and ugly-faced him, pointing to *another* backhouse all the way over on the other side of the schoolyard. Now the front of his pants were damp and his teeth were clenched with trying to hold. A long time to the other backhouse and unbutton the big bone buttons that wadded in the double thick of wet cloth. Too late. When he came out of the backhouse, he knew that he was only to be sad, very sad for the wood-day.

There was no one in the schoolyard now. He went back to the big building, opening the door that was closed, as he knew he must . . .

When he was let go at last from the building, the light was long and golden and sad with its going. He was surprised and confused at the length of the light. Didn't he take all the day's pain with a strong face, never weeping once, never running away? Wasn't that enough, without the day being used away besides? In spite of all he could do, his eyes filled. He looked about, trying to find some secret place where he might creep away and cry . . .

There was a cart coming towards the place from down the road. He watched the light catch its metal now and then, and once or twice it was overtaken by its own dust. A terrifying hope began. It came up and beat inside his body. His father, dead these long light-passing times, was coming back. His father-mother-farm-life was coming back to take him away, to take him home, to forgive him. He began to run in circles, unable to contain his joy and his gratitude. Then he stood humbly, as a person does at any miracle. Never had his father been so powerful or so straight, never so different and so much the same.

Abel was standing motionless as the cart came on. His father saw him and raised a hand and then smiled at him. They had forgiven him. He got up into the cart before it stopped and they turned and left the bad things behind him. The day of pain was over.

When they came back to the farm, his mother asked him about Uuuuuu and he smiled and nodded because it was over and he had lived through it and came back into the season of living things, and into their forgiveness again. It was only when his mother set his clothes of that day carefully on the chair again did he realize what his punishment was to be. Tomorrow also. The day after that. He stopped breathing; there was a pushing in his throat.

That night, he lay staring out at the dark sky, unable to cry himself to sleep. In front of the window the maple tree moved. He felt angry that he had been in this bed this morning, knowing so little. Beside him lay his younger brother, sleeping. He began to shake the bed to wake up the little boy who was taking the days so easily. The boy turned and slept on. Once, Abel knew, he had trusted like that. Once, he, too, had been good. For a while he watched the night and the moon in balance on the slender tips of branches.

From that day on, the time, which before had been a long measure, was now hung for him in endless strings of five and two. His mother began to wait for him with pencil and paper, and sometimes he wrote words there, but only the ones he had learned in school. He did not understand what they meant to be, and he never understood her when she tried to make them important to him. She was eager, somehow, and then angry, and finally, only sad. It was his fault, for which he was being punished. Soon she got tired and stopped.

From *In this Sign*

Edith and Monica, staying at the Hotel du Lac, observe one of the long-term residents, Mme de Bonneuil, being visited by her son and daughter-in-law.

The sound of wheels on gravel brought their heads round. Mme de Bonneuil, her pug face creased into a smile, was struggling to her feet. A car door banged, and a man walked jauntily into the garden, followed by a woman in a red dress, the spikes of her high-heeled sandals plunging into the lawn. '*Eh bien, maman,*' cried the man, falsely cheery. Kisses were exchanged.

'Poor old trout,' said Monica, her tone very slightly lower. 'She lives for that son. She'd do anything for him. And he comes to see her once a month, takes her out in the car, brings her back, and forgets her.'

'Why is she here?' asked Edith.

Monica shrugged. 'His idea entirely. He considers her manners too rustic for her to be allowed to live under the same roof as that frightful wife of his who, incidentally, started life as a hairdresser before snaffling her first husband. This one's her second. Mme de Bonneuil had a beautiful house near the French border: it's quite a good family, incidentally. Naturally, the daughter-in-law wanted the house to herself. So the old girl had to go. She can't stand the wife, of course. Despises her. Quite right. She lives here because she doesn't want to see the son unhappy.'

'How do you know all this?' asked Edith,' startled and impressed.

'She told me,' said Monica, inhaling from another cigarette.

'I have never heard her say a single word,' mused Edith.

'Well, it's difficult for her.' To Edith's enquiring glance Monica replied, 'She's stone deaf. What a life.'

. . .

Mme de Bonneuil, her smile now tinged with anxiety, sat while her son and daughter-in-law discussed matters common only to themselves in loud voices which she could not hear. Finally, her son, responding to a cocked head, and an *'On s'en va?'* from his wife, stood up with alacrity and prepared to leave. His wife offered her cheek to the mother-in-law and tripped off to the car. Mme de Bonneuil attempted to retain her son but the car horn sounded, and *'J'arrive,'* he called, kissing his mother noisily on both cheeks. Mme de Bonneuil remained standing on the terrace, gazing in the direction of her vanished son, until the silence in which she spent her days was palpable even to Edith . . .

From *Hotel du Lac*

> Musical people are so absurdly unreasonable. They always want one to be perfectly dumb at the very moment when one is longing to be absolutely deaf.
>
> Oscar Wilde

*Nate Twomey, the coffin maker, at home with Bertha,
his widowed sister.*

The flesh of the rabbit fell away moistly from the bones. But in the middle of eating he had to raise his handkerchief to his left eye again and again, where the chip of wood had flown into it that morning, leaving it watery and sore. So that when Bertha spoke to him, he could not see her face and so missed what she was saying. He read her lips more easily than those of anyone else, she had only to mumble and he knew, for it was she who had first taught him, and shown him how to write, too, she had been more patient with his deafness and dumbness than either of their parents, who were uneasy, never knowing what he might be thinking, and frightened of being judged and blamed by the rest of the village. There had been one other child, also a boy, who had died, but he had been quite sound, they felt bitter it was Nate who grew up in place of him.

Bertha Twomey waited. She always ate her own meal alone, after her brother had gone back to the workshop, and now, she stood beside the wooden kitchen table until he had finished wiping his eyes.

'You damaged yourself then, haven't you?'

He pointed to his eye.

'Splinters. You want to be more careful – putting your head too close to that bench, that's what. I told you before about that.'

He shook his head but his eye was watering freely, he had to wipe it again and then she insisted on looking at it more closely. It was bloodshot and swimming with tears. In the end, she got the splinter out with the twisted corner of a clean handkerchief. 'You be more careful what you're doing in future, Nate Twomey.' He grinned, nodding at her. They had always been like this together, she treating him like a child, while still knowing that he was not a fool, just because he was deaf and dumb. She was two years older but she had been the first one to push him out, not so long after she had learned to walk herself, they were very close.

From 'Halloran's Child', in *A Bit of Singing and Dancing*

MARTIN CRUZ SMITH 1942–

Three bodies, shot dead, are found buried under snow in Moscow's
Gorky Park. Detective Pasha investigates.

'It occurred to me' – Pasha tried to be matter-of-fact – 'that maybe
something besides snow covered the sound of the gunshots. After
wasting most of the day with the food vendors, I go and talk to the
little old woman who plays the records over the loudspeakers for
the skating in the park during the winter. She has a little room in
the building at the Krimsky Val entrance. I ask, "Do you play any
loud records?" She says, "Only quiet records for skating." I ask,
"Do you have a program of music you follow every day?" She says,
"Programs are for television, I only play records for skating, quiet
records played by a simple laborer, the same as I have since the war
when I was in the artillery. I earned my job honestly," she says,
"for my disability." I say, "That's not my concern, I just want to
know the order of the records you play." "The right order," she
says. "I start at the top of the pile and work my way down, and
when there are no more records I know it's time to go home."
"Show me," I say. The old woman brings out a stack of fifteen
records. They're even numbered one to fifteen. I was thinking the
shooting probably took place toward the end of the day, and so I
work from the back. Number fifteen, sure enough, is from *Swan
Lake*. Number fourteen, you want to guess? The *1812 Overture*.
Cannons, bells, the works. Finally, I'm getting smart. Why should
the records have to be numbered? I hold the record in front of my
mouth and ask her, "How loud do you play the records?" She just
looks; she hasn't heard a thing. The old woman is deaf, that's her
disability, and that's who they have playing the records in Gorky
Park!'

From *Gorky Park*

171

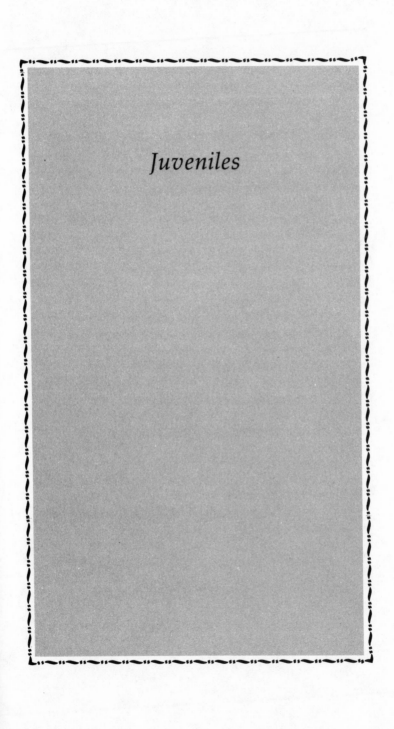

Juveniles

Three survivors of the 'Great Blast' have made a home together.

There were three of them, Wystan, Bridget, and Hadrian, and they were a most unusual household. They lived all by themselves in a hut at the edge of a great wood, and the eldest was blind, the second was lame, and the third could not hear a single word, even if you shouted . . .

No one bothered that Hadrian was deaf, and often the two elder ones spoke to him just as they spoke to each other so that he lost a certain amount of general conversation. But he was very sharp. He picked up a good deal of what they said, as he often boasted. But when there was something special that his two elders wanted him to understand, they said it very particularly clearly with their mouths and spelt it out with their hands . . .

Occasionally a Straggler from the Waste would come prying into the wood to see what he could seize or steal. Then the three children had to look out. Their hut was concealed behind a thicket off the main path, and most of the Stragglers with their torn clothing and wild appearance passed the place by . . .

But this time Hadrian was in a spot where the trees were sparse and there was no hiding-place. He was just beginning to turn and run when a hand seized his collar and twisted him round.

'Who the dickens are you?' said a voice, which of course Hadrian could not hear, being deaf. And he couldn't see either because the hand had pulled up the back of his jersey with such a jerk that it covered his face in front.

'Answer!' said the voice. Now if Hadrian had been able to hear, he would have noticed that the voice, for all its authority, had that curious broken sound between bass and treble that belongs to a boy in his teens. And he would not have been so frightened. As it was, he continued to believe that he had been caught by a tramp. He held himself very still and then suddenly let his body go limp and his arms swing over his head. Immediately he slipped to the ground, leaving his jersey in his astonished captor's hand, and made off like a flash.

175

But ... he had not a clumsy older man to escape. The young invader to the wood dodged and sprinted just as cleverly as Hadrian, who without thinking had bolted off towards home. Hadrian stumbled and felt himself caught again. He rolled over and found himself looking into the face of a handsome boy dressed in a torn red shirt with a rucksack on his back.

'Now tell me who you are, or I'll bash you to bits,' said the unknown boy. Hadrian said nothing because he had heard nothing and was too dazed to see what the boy's mouth was saying.

'Speak up, you misery,' cried the boy.

'I'd let him go if I were you,' said a voice behind him. 'He can't hear you, you know; he's deaf.' Wystan and Bridget had come running out at the sound of the chase.

'I'm not hurting him; you can see that for yourselves,' said the boy grumpily.

'Well actually I can't, you know,' said Wystan. 'I'm blind.'

'Blind! Deaf! And I suppose you're ...' He turned angrily to the girl who stood beside Wystan. 'Oh I'm sorry,' he added, hesitating. 'I didn't see.'

'It's all right,' said Bridget. 'Of course you didn't. How do you do.' And she limped forward with a hand outstretched.

From *Into the Forest*

*In the year 1852 Davy Halladay, his younger brother John Willie,
and their father, are trapped underground in a mining disaster.*

The water rushed at them. It was as if the floor of the pit had
opened and the sea were pouring in. Davy Halladay couldn't
believe it was water; even in the light of the swinging lamps the
top of it still looked like the floor of the pit because it was covered
with coal dust; only the dead chilliness around his legs, then his
thighs and now his waist told him it was water all right. He was
yelling, to his father, 'Da! Da! where's John Willie? Da! John Willie
.. he's gone.' ...

He'd always had the idea that had John Willie had the right food
he wouldn't have continued to be deaf and dumb. He had the idea
that the right food would have loosened something at the back of
his tongue and in his ears, for he had never heard of rich people's
children being deaf and dumb ... If only his body had grown at
the same rate as his hair his brother, Davy knew, would have been
a giant, not an undersized deaf mute, not 'Halladay's idiot' as he
was called by many.

But John Willie, Davy knew, was no idiot. Behind the silence of
his tongue and the deafness of his ears there was a knowing. But it
was only he himself who seemed to recognize the knowing; even
his father looked upon his younger son as an idiot, not simply
because he was unable to communicate as an ordinary boy would,
but because he was puny in strength.

At nine years old John Willie should have been able to earn a
shilling a day down the pit. Boys of his age did horses' work;
where the roofs were too low to allow for the passage of the pit
ponies the boys were harnessed with an iron chain between their
legs to the bogies, and, going on all-fours, dragged them through
the low passages. But John Willie was no good for that kind of
work, he was no good for nothing, his father said.

Although John Willie came down the pit with his father and
Davy, he wasn't on the pay roll; he was allowed to come down with

177

them by courtesy of the butty, and this had come about only through the insistence of Davy, not of his father. Davy had dared to stand up to his father and say he wouldn't go down unless he could take John Willie along with him, for to leave him up above meant leaving him to the mercy of the villagers. Some were all right towards him but others, those who were apt to believe in omens and signs, pelted him whenever he crossed their path.

Mrs Coxon's lot were the worst. There were ten Coxons and whenever possible they would make sport of John Willie. It was their Sunday game, the only day in the week when they could play when they weren't working in the fields, or down the mine, and if there wasn't much to do they hunted out John Willie and, making a circle round him, pushed him from one to the other.

His da and Mr Coxon had had a stand up fight one Sunday. That was the only time Davy had really been proud of his da, for on that day his da had defended John Willie with his fists for the first time.

But now where was his da? And where was he? Where were they?

From Our John Willie

Johnnie Cass, a battered twelve year old, whose hearing is severely damaged by his step-father's brutality, flounders at school and encounters hostility in the playground.

What was the question? What was he supposed to say? He never knew.

'You'll have to stay behind and write it out. Do you hear me?'

He didn't. But despairingly, he nodded. He stayed behind.

Sometimes they showed him what to write, and he wrote it – beautifully. He had strong, well-formed writing, fluent and easy. He had taught himself to write, from endless blackboard copying which was supposed to be a punishment. But it was like drawing. He enjoyed it.

But if they didn't tell him what to say, how could he write it? He didn't understand education. It seemed a mystifying process. What exactly did they want him to do? He never found out.

All the same, he quite liked staying in. It was better than going out. The playground was terrifying. The shouting got louder and louder. His ears hurt like fire. Gangs of boys set on him, chanting things at him. He could see their red mouths opening and shutting. Yapping at him, like dogs.

'Johnnie Dumbo! Johnnie Dumbo!
Hasn't got a single Crumbo!'

The circle of faces bounced round at him, advancing like a wall of pale balloons.

'Johnnie Dim
Hasn't got a glim!

Johnnie Moo (That was those eyes again)
Hasn't got a clue!

Johnnie Cass
Bottom of the class!

Pea-brain Johnnie,
Flea-brain Johnnie!
Johnnie Dimbo
Lives in limbo!'

From *Johnnie Alone*

Pippa, at the age of six, fractured her skull and suffered multiple injuries in an accident. After many operations and a prolonged stay in hospital her doctor talks to her before sending her home.

'What do you remember best?'

Her lips repeated his words and she thought for a moment.

'Daddy r-reading s-stories an' M-mummy p-playing the p-piano. An' B-brownie when she w-whistled – you h-had to g-go AT ONCE. An' early in the m-morning the b-birds outside – all of them s-singing at once.'

She held up her hand with her fingers spread out.

'Show m-me how m-many d-days an' I w-will be h-home,' she asked.

He counted, bending her thin little fingers one by one into the palm of her hand. 'Thursday, Friday, Saturday. Three more days and you will be home again.' She drew in her breath in a long, quivering sigh.

'Yes,' she murmured happily. 'Three more d-days and I w-will h-hear them all again. D-daddy reading, an' Brownie, an' the b-birds s-singing in the m-morning . . .'

The doctor pulled her close to him so that she would not see the shock her words had given him. Throughout her long illness he had been her only link with reality and in her pain and helplessness she had clung to him. He thought that he understood all her fears and anxieties, but the realisation that for all these months she had associated her deafness only with her stay in hospital appalled him. Never had he felt so powerless to help anyone.

At last he made himself lean back in his chair and look at her. She was smiling up at him, her eyes bright and a faint colour in her pale cheeks. He took her hands in his and spoke slowly and firmly, shaking his head to emphasise his words.

'Pippa, you will not be able to hear when you go home on Saturday.'

Again her lips moved, repeating his words, then she gave him a patient, understanding little smile. The smile one might give to a child who had not quite understood what it has been told.

'B-but I c-can always h-hear at h-home. It is only in the h-hospital I c-can't.'

He could only shake his head.

For a moment she stared at him, then her hands became tight fists in his and he felt her body stiffen. His heart ached as he watched the colour drain from her face.

'Pippa, you must understand.' He tried to unclinch her hands but she pulled them away and put them behind her back. He touched the bandage around her head.

'When your head is quite better you will hear again.'

But she persisted.

'A-at h-home I always h-hear,' she whispered piteously; 'at h-home I w-will.'

He could feel her going from him as surely as if she were walking from the room. He made one final effort and put his hand under her chin, turning her face to make her look at him.

'Will you do something for me?'

'I d-don't k-know.'

'Please, Pippa,' he begged. 'You must watch and listen all the time.'

But she dropped her head and stared at her clenched fists.

For a while it had been just like really hearing again – talking to him and remembering. But the noise was back in her ears, blowing softly, insistently. And when she watched his face she could only see his lips moving.

The book ends with Pippa being able to hear Brownie's whistle again.

Pippa stopped suddenly, her head on one side like a small bright bird. For a second she hesitated.

'We're wanted!' she shouted.

In stunned silence they watched as she turned and raced joyfully back along the road to her father's outstretched arms.

From *Robbie's Mob*

181

'Tuppence', a moorland pony, helps Martin to come to terms with his deafness.

The pony came to the edge of the ramp. Its head was up, its ears were sharp. It looked around to the orchard, the shippens, the farmhouse. It stared a long time at the moor which rose above the farm.

Harvey stood on one side of the lorry, Jane on the other. He was the pony-farmer from whom the pony had been bought. She was his ten-year-old daughter. They had brought it to the Manninghams of Shepherds Hill. Now they watched to see what would happen.

Nathan, the farm-hand, nudged the halter. For a moment the pony resisted. Then it put one foot on the straw which covered the ramp. One foot meant two feet. Nathan kept it going until suddenly the pony was out of the lorry and in the orchard lane. It turned quickly, trying to see everything at once. Nathan patted its neck. Then he looked to Martin, waiting for the boy to show a sign.

Martin was eleven years old. He guessed that this was supposed to be a big occasion, that his father had planned it carefully, hoping to surprise him. Martin knew that many boys of his age would be delighted and grateful. But the delight was not there. Neither was the gratitude.

He could not forget that he was different now. Different from other boys who had been his friends at school; different from Jane who was his only friend on the moor. He could not forget that he had been made different by this silence which had come suddenly bewildering him and so frightening his parents that they didn' know what to do.

The pony was the idea of parents who didn't know what to do. I was a gift. He was supposed to go hunting, to compete i gymkhanas. He was supposed to pretend that nothing had happened, that he could take his place among other boys and girls Martin thought his parents didn't understand. He didn't want t

de, to hunt, to pretend that nothing had happened. He didn't
ant to try because he didn't believe it. He knew how different he
ad become. Now he felt his parents watching. His mother was
miling, hiding her anxiety, begging him to be what they wanted
im to be. His father's eyes were begging, too. But behind the
egging was a tightening impatience.

Martin didn't glance to Jane. He didn't glance to Harvey, who
as boasting about the pony. He glanced to Nathan, hoping the
rizzled old farm-hand would understand.

Nathan held the halter, stroking the pony's face. The pony was a
Dartmoor. It had been foaled on the moor and Harvey had brought
in and chosen it for breaking. Jane had helped in the breaking.
he'd been helping her father since she was six.

Now Mr Manningham had bought it, trying to please his son.
Martin knew what they wanted him to say.

'Thank you, it's lovely.'

The words were in his head, but when he tried to speak the
ords wouldn't come. It had often been like this. He was afraid of
peaking, of feeling the effort in his throat, then of hearing
othing. Not to hear your own voice when you speak. That was
omething he hadn't grown used to yet. He looked at his mother.
Her smile encouraged him to risk it. Finally he said, 'Thank you,
's very nice.' Then he shot Jane a glance, defying her to laugh
ecause his voice was wrong.

Once he had seen a play, and in the play there had been a comic
haracter, very funny. This comic character had cupped a hand
ehind his ear and said, 'Eh?', showing that he was deaf. The
udience had roared, making deafness a very funny thing.

He had not cared then. That had been before the accident, and
eafness had not mattered. It had been only something that
appened to others, usually to the old. But now it was different.
Now it mattered. Now it had happened to him.

His father came near. Martin did not hear the footsteps, but he
elt his father coming. There was a tremor of fear, not because he
as afraid of his father but because he was ashamed and resentful.
He guessed that deafness made him seem a fool.

He thought that his father would speak, speaking loudly the way
eople do to the deaf. He could always tell when his father was
houting. The impatience in the eyes gave it away. But this time his

183

father did not shout. Mr Manningham held out his hand, showin
Martin the hand so he would not be shocked by a sudden touc
The hand asked to be trusted and Martin went with him towar
the pony.

The book ends with the birth of a foal to Tuppence.

He touched the foal with one hand and scratched the mare with th
other. He was not laughing, but there was laughter in his hear
Martin did not feel resentful of what had happened to his ear
He did not feel different and shut in. He didn't suspect all th
world of laughing at him.

He felt rich.

From *Martin Rides the Mo*

Long ago in ancient times, Sadhi, the son of Reuben, Prince of Canaan, and of Thamar, his wife, has become deaf without speech following illness at the age of five. His frustration and anger which neither his parents nor Caltah, his nurse, can control make him subject to violent and destructive tempers. In search of a cure he is entrusted to the care of the wise and learned Hekhti, who keeps him isolated from his family and remains unmoved by Sadhi's tantrums for three long days and nights.

The Chief Royal Architect had his own apartments in the immense rambling warren of the Palace. Caltah carried Sadhi into Hekhti's presence, and left him there. At first he made no attempt to escape, but seemed overawed, and sat where he had been placed on a pile of cushions in the centre of the floor, and looked round him. Like a small animal he was sensing the atmosphere of his surroundings.

Hekhti's main room was large, high and rectangular, its ceiling supported by the conventional columns topped with lotus buds. The floor was black and white inlay of some stone which felt warm to the soles of Sadhi's feet. The room's three entrances – to right and left and at one end – were covered by hangings of plain white linen. Decoration was confined to the ceiling, where bee and plant, vulture and serpent, all symbols of the Two Lands, were repeated in gold and turquoise and lapis again and again.

Sadhi lowered his gaze to where Hekhti himself sat crosslegged upon the floor. At his side was a low table, covered with plans. He was writing on a length of papyrus, but looked up occasionally at his small patient, smiled, and returned to work.

The silence, the austerity, Hekhti's presence: Sadhi summed them up and didn't like them. Pining and frail he might be, but he could still summon up the nervous energy that some sick people show. He was suddenly on his feet, darting for the nearest entrance. He grabbed on the linen hangings and pulled them apart. Outside stood one of the King's Bodyguard, who smiled pleasantly but raised his spear to a horizontal position and barred Sadhi's path.

The child stared, backed away. He wheeled and charged across the room, only to fall into the arms of another guard outside the second entrance. Sadhi made an inarticulate sound of rage and charged the third entrance even faster – with the same result. All the time Hekhti paid him no attention, and continued to work.

So it went on: Sadhi didn't give up easily. He feinted towards one entrance and made for another. He almost succeeded in twisting out between one soldier's feet. Yet each time he was caught, and gently prodded back into the room again. His rage mounted. It was impossible to show quite what he felt – his thin chest heaved, he gasped, he pummelled, he fought. At last he expressed his sense of outrage by kicking and kicking at one of the eternally smiling soldiers, and then retreated to the cushions, lay on his face, and thrashed with all his limbs as though hoping to break the floor.

Presently his physical condition told on him. His frenzy gave way to stillness, except for an occasional heaving sob. Then even that ceased. After some while he sat up again, his hands pressed over his eyes. He looked a pathetic, beaten object, but there was something about the way he sat – Hekhti, eyeing him thoughtfully, rose, put down his papyrus, and picked up a jug of fruit juice from the table by him. He filled a carved cup, bore it to Sadhi's side, placed one hand on the child's shoulder and, when the guarded position relaxed very slightly, offered him the cup.

Sadhi's thin brows slanted downwards and then together in a frown. Sadhi's eyes peered upward like a nervous and suspicious oryx's. He drew back an arm and struck the cup away from him so forcibly that it fell from Hekhti's hand and shattered to pieces on the floor. A stream of golden liquid spread across the patterned black and white.

Hekhti showed no reaction – but waited quietly, his hand still on Sadhi's shoulder. After a second's scowling into that impassive face Sadhi shrugged out from out under the architect's hand and struck wildly in the direction of his mouth. Hekhti was too quick for him, and moved aside. Impetus carried the child forward on to his face. Before he had time flailing at the floor he was picked up and returned firmly to the cushions. While he was still sitting there, dazed with surprise, Hekhti returned to the room's far end, reseated himself, and clapped his hand for Amrat, who came unning to clear up the spilled juice and remove the shattered cup. Vhen the room was silent once more, Hekhti resumed his work.

Sadhi stayed where he was, and did nothing for some while, but is tension grew and grew till it was unbearable along with his atred and frustration . . .

Hekhti was carefully inscribing on his papyrus when Sadhi harged at the table like a small bull. He banged into it heavily, urt himself, and leaned sobbing against the top; then, with one weep of both arms, he sent everything – plans, writing materials, ruit juice – cascading to destruction on the floor. Hekhti paid no ttention whatever, but continued writing until something like a niniature cyclone hurled itself upon him from behind. He let fall is scroll, turned, and caught Sadhi by the wrists to lift him ffortlessly and carry him back towards the cushions. Violent ttempts to escape from them were restrained without violence of ny sort. Meanwhile Amrat, who had heard the crash, re-entered to leal with the resultant chaos. Once Sadhi's hysterical fighting had uietened down, Hekhti returned to his writing, ignoring an ccasional exaggerated sob . . .

Then, quite suddenly, half-way through the fourth day, Sadhi's letermination crumbled. He had been raging round the room all norning showing reserves of nervous energy which seemed in- redible . . . He had hurled cushions, sobbed, attacked just as efore. But around midday when the sun stood at full strength bove the Palace, and the heat was infernal, and the shadows of olumns black upon the floor, Sadhi gave a great sigh of exhaus- ion. He raised his eyes, which now looked enormous, and gazed at is impassive tormentor. His glance travelled over Hekhti's face as hough seeking some kind of a crack in that relentless impassivity. here was none. No evidence of strain, of fright, of possible giving p. He knew at last that no one would bring Thamar here with altah, nor let him free.

Of course he could punish them all by starving himself until he lied. One part of him – no, more, a *great* part – wanted to do just hat, and watch them wring their hands and be unhappy around is bed. But where *were* his mother and father – and where was the errifying pleasure of rejecting life if he couldn't see their alarm and njoy inflicting pain on them? There would only be this stranger to it by him, kindly compassionate but not sorry enough – no, not *nearly* sorry enough! – to make it all worth while. He glowered across the room at the man who couldn't be beaten, who wouldn' raise a finger to stop him going alone into the darkness of which when he really thought about it, he was so very much afraid . . Amrat was just bringing in the midday meal, and looked at Sadhi beckoning to him. The child took a few wavering steps forward and received the full warmth of Hekhti's encouraging smile. Just to eat once meant nothing, Sadhi thought. He could refuse again any time he chose. In a very dignified manner he approached. Hekhti made a simple, downward gesture. Sadhi sat. Then he put out a hesitant hand towards the food.

But, to his utter amazement, Hekhti prevented him by taking hold of his hand in a firm grip and tapping twice on it. Sadhi looked at him, very puzzled. Hekhti released his hand and gave him the bowl; as he started to eat, removed it from him, took his hand, tapped on it as before, and again handed him the bowl Sadhi's ferocious scowl began to form. He was almost ready to start throwing things, but he was so hungry by now and the food smelled too enticing! In spite of himself he ate, casting suspicious sidelong glances at his companion.

When Amrat approached to serve them with a light wine, Sadhi snatched greedily at the cup, but again Hekhti intercepted him. He doubled Sadhi's hand into a fist, closing the child's fingers inward and holding them there. It was done twice and then he was allowed the cup. Quite suddenly Sadhi got the message. That gesture meant 'drink' just as the first had meant 'food' or 'eat'. Someone had managed to break through his lack of communication and the awful silence of the outer world! He was so surprised by the blinding revelation that you could actually speak *without* speaking that he gave Hekhti a wondering smile.

Something of Reuben's charm appeared on his pinched features Hekhti was more moved by that pathetic smile than he had been by anything in the preceding days. He put his arm around the child to draw him to his side, and kissed him on the forehead as Reuben would have done. Sadhi stiffened. Then, lulled by a strange sense of confidence in this man he couldn't make afraid, and by the pleasure of a full stomach, he leaned heavily against Hekhti and went straight to sleep. For a long while Hekhti sat there holding the child's fragile body in his arms. He sat as still as he always did, and

188

there was very little expression on his features except one of faint surprise.*

From *The Bright and Morning Star*

* Hekhti's 'taming' of Sadhi bears a strong resemblance to Annie Sullivan's treatment of the young Helen Keller, who was just as wild and frustrated as Sadhi, when Annie Sullivan became her governess and teacher.

Deafness is a disability without pathos.

One ought at once to admit to deafness. One seldom does as one ought.

The gulf between the speaking and the signing deaf and again between the life-long and the lately deafened can be deep and wide.

The disabled have been given a built-in, ready packed objective which is always present, a definite impediment to get the better of. Like the prospect of hanging, it concentrates the mind wonderfully.

David Wright

David's family has moved to enable him to attend a school for deaf children. Michael, his new neighbour, befriends him but cannot persuade other boys to do the same.

'I can't stand the way he looks at me. It gives me the creeps.'

'Why?' asked Michael.

'I don't know. It just does.'

'But he's got to look. It's the only way he has of knowing anything.'

'I've nothing against people like him, but I just don't want to have anything to do with them.'

'Would you keep out of the way of someone who is blind?'

'Of course not. That's different.'

'Why?'

'Well, it's terrible to be blind.'

'It's terrible to be totally deaf.'

'But it's not the same.'

'Why?'

'Well, they're dumb, stupid, simple. They're not normal, almost loony and I don't like loonies.'

'But can't you see,' burst out Michael, 'that's just where you're wrong? Oh, I know David sometimes looks like a dim-wit – and acts like one; but if he could hear, he'd be just like us. He could talk, and read, and learn, and – oh, everything!'

Peter however was not to be convinced, and came back to his first point, adding:

'I still think you're a bit soft about his being deaf.'

From *David in Silence*

Shane learns from his sister Shelley that his new friend is 'deaf'.

Shelley spent the interval between five o'clock and tea-time polishing her nails and wishing it were Saturday. During the meal she brought up the subject of clothes, for the tenth time that week.

'Mum, this new boy wants to take me to the dance, and I honestly don't have a thing to wear—'

'What boy?' demanded Mr Halliday.

'Graham Calder. You know – that new family in Kennedy Place. His brother is a friend of Shane's.'

'You're supposed to ask our permission before you go dancing with perfectly strange boys,' said her father. 'We don't know anything about this Graham.'

'But we do, Dad. He's seventeen, and he's from Melbourne, and he's working at the Southdale Service Station. And he has a younger brother who's deaf.'

Shane, who had been eating steadily and silently in the hope of being first to the television after tea, paused in mid-bite.

'Who said? The only brother he's got is Glen.'

'I know that, silly. And Glen's deaf – Graham told me.'

'He isn't,' Shane insisted, pushing away his plate. 'He can't be. I ought to know – I've been friends with him for a whole week.'

'Why should Graham make up a thing like that?' Shelley demanded. 'It must be true.'

She returned tenaciously to the topic of a new dress.

Shane didn't listen; he had been studying the T.V. programmes guide under cover of the tablecloth, but now he let it slide to the floor. As a rule he chose to look forward rather than backward, and to accept life as it came, so it was quite an effort to recall everything he knew of Glen Calder, in the light of what Shelley had said.

Shane and Shelley had had a great-aunt who was deaf; he vaguely remembered going to visit her in an old people's home, and Shelley had been overcome with embarrassment at having to shout throughout the conversation. Shane had felt sorry for the old

191

lady, who seemed so cut-off in all respects from the everyday world, and he had pleased her by going up and speaking right into her ear, in his best cricket-field voice.

But Glen wasn't like that. He didn't expect his companions to shout at him, and he answered questions like anyone else, except that—

'I suppose he does miss things now and then,' said Shane, more to himself than to his family. 'And he stares at whoever's doing the talking, all the time.'

'Poor boy,' remarked Mrs Halliday sympathetically. 'It must be such a handicap.'

Shane didn't like that word, either. It suggested that Glen was some sort of cripple, or one of those unfortunate children who went to the special school in Acacia Park, because they couldn't learn anything in ordinary classes. And Shane knew that Glen was as normal as himself, much more intelligent in fact. He hated the idea of his friend being branded as 'different'.

From *The Nothing Place*

Edmund (alias 'Mundo'), deafened by illness at the age of seven, is bewildered by the changes made by his loss of hearing.

I kept trying to be the same, but everything else was different. Cups and saucers didn't clatter. The kettle huffed and puffed without a sound. My parents moved their lips in conversation with one another, but not a word emerged. What they wanted to say to me, they awkwardly tried to mime.

There was something else too, that I found harder to understand. I had never realized before how much my ears had told me where things were, where I was myself. When I picked up my cup, I didn't feel sure that I was holding it. When I put it down, it was with an unexpected jolt. Sound, I was discovering, is a gauge to so much more than hearing. I wasn't sure that I could smell my toast, or even taste it. I wasn't sure that my feet touched the ground. I started to shake my head, upset by the increasing sense of unreality. Ridiculously, I thought that if I shook it hard enough, I might shake off the silence. My parents looked horribly alarmed. Then I accidentally knocked over the jug.

I saw it smash into pieces, splattering everything with milk, including my father's suit. It hadn't made a sound.

I was filled with a sense of horror. It was like a ghost jug in a ghost room with a ghost mother and father. I was like a ghost boy!

His discovery of sound and of the 'weather-child' in a fantasy world 'on the other side of silence' gradually heals the shock of his deafness.

I looked and I listened, as hard as I could, but all I could hear was the silence. In the shadowy stillness, before the lights went on in the houses, I discovered that silence has an echo, that silence, in a way, resounds.

I thought: If this silence was deep enough, and I listened hard enough, I might pass through to its other side. And on the other

193

side of silence, who knows what I might find? Perhaps another world of sound, which only I could hear? I would be like the child in the story who goes through the looking glass, or the one who finds a secret door.

Resounding, sounding silence! It echoed inside my head. Listen! Listen ever so hard! What can there be to hear? . . .

'Why can I hear you when I can't hear anything else?'

'*Can't* you hear anything else?'

'No. Not a sound.'

'Not a sound?'

'No. Not car engines or voices or factory hooters or church bell or aeroplanes or hammers or squeaking or scraping or—' I would have gone on and on if the weather-child hadn't stopped me.

'Oh *those* things!' he said. 'Those are only noises—'

'—or music or marbles or birds or singing. I can't even hear my own voice!' I shouted, at the top of it.

And then I realized something else: whenever I talked to the weather-child I *could* hear my own voice! But he was talking now. 'Those are the things that you listen to with your ears. Listen to other things instead.'

'*What* other things shall I listen to and what *with* but my ears?'

'Everything *but* your ears.'

'I don't know what you mean,' I shouted, exasperated with the effort of trying to understand . . .

And he told me. He told me about all the underground sounds, about humming and drumming and throbbing, from subterranean caverns and streams; about twisting winding hollows, tunnelling to the centre of the earth. He told me about a music so deep and dark, from that very still middle, that it isn't so much heard as felt. He said the earth was veined with sound.

He told me about a music so high and far that it echoes from star to star, to the edges of outer space, and resounds from sun to sun and moon to moon, coming back to the earth again.

And he told me last of all about the music of the weather.

Between the deep dark chords of the earth music and the high light notes of the sky music, the weather plays its symphonies, with sounds of light and shade, sun and rain, calm and storm, hot and cold, to the rhythms of the changing seasons. He made it sound all so beautiful.

'I don't hear this music with my *ears*, I listen with all of me. I become the music. The music plays on me.'

'So you can be what you hear, as well as what you see,' I said.

From *Mundo and the Weather-Child**

* This book was written when Joyce Dunbar's own son Ben began to go deaf at the age of five. By giving him a hero to identify with, she hoped to help him come to terms with his deafness. 'I'd tried to reconcile Ben to his deafness by explaining it to him in an adult way, but it's very difficult to give meanings to children with explanations. The way to reach them is through stories. The way to appeal to people's deepest sense of understanding is through the imagination.' Joyce Dunbar is partially deaf herself and experienced great difficulty in accepting her deafness until her husband helped her to do so at the age of twenty-three. 'I thought, if he can accept me, I can accept me.'

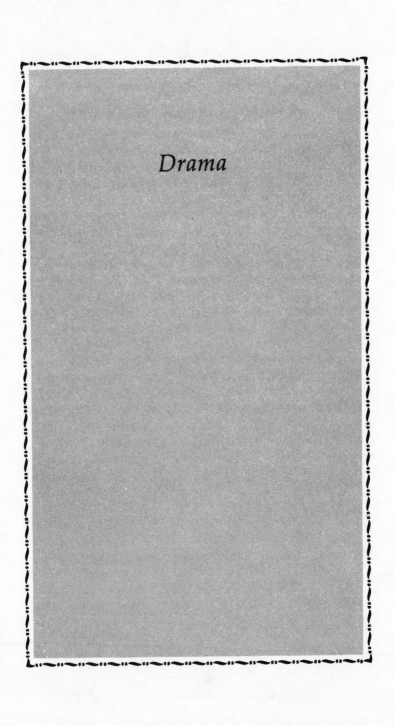

Drama

Was Caesar deaf in one ear?

CAESAR: Such men as he be never at heart's ease
    Whiles they behold a greater than themselves,
    And therefore are they very dangerous.
    I rather tell thee what is to be fear'd
    Than what I fear, for always I am Caesar.
    Come on my right hand, for this ear is deaf,
    And tell me truly what thou thinks't of him.

From *Julius Caesar*, Act 1

Aged Aegeon pleads for recognition.

AEGEON: Not know my voice! O, time's extremity,
    Hast thou so crack'd and splitted my poor tongue
    In seven short years, that here my only son
    Knows not my feeble key of untun'd cares?
    Though now this grained face of mine be hid
    In sap-consuming winter's drizzled snow,
    And all the conduits of my blood froze up,
    Yet hath my night of life some memory,
    My wasting lamps some fading glimmer left,
    My dull deaf ears a little use to hear:
    All these old witnesses, I cannot err,
    Tell me thou art my son Antipholus.

From *The Comedy of Errors*, Act 5

Annie Sullivan after a long train journey arrives at the station for the Keller homestead in Tuscumbia, Alabama to take up her employment as Helen's governess. Kate and James, Helen's mother and brother, welcome her.

ANNIE: You – live far from town, Mrs Keller?

KATE: Only a mile.

ANNIE: Well. I suppose I can wait one more mile. But don't be surprised if I get out and push the horse!

KATE: Helen's waiting for you, too. There's been such a bustle in the house, she expects something, heaven knows what. (*Now she voices part of her doubt, not as such but* ANNIE *understands it.*) I expected – a desiccated spinster. You're very young.

ANNIE (*resolutely*): Oh, you should have seen me when I left Boston. I got much older on this trip.

KATE: I mean, to teach anyone as difficult as Helen.

ANNIE: I mean to try. They can't put you in jail for trying!

KATE: Is it possible, even? To teach a deaf-blind child half of what an ordinary child learns – has that ever been done?

ANNIE: Half?

KATE: A tenth.

ANNIE (*reluctantly*): No. (KATE's *face loses its remaining hope, still appraising her youth.*) Dr Howe* did wonders, but – an ordinary child? No, never. But then I thought when I was going over his reports – (*She indicates the one in her hand.*) – he never treated them like ordinary children. More like – eggs everyone was afraid would break.

KATE (*a pause*): May I ask how old are you?

ANNIE: Well, I'm not in my teens, you know! I'm twenty.

KATE: All of twenty.

ANNIE (*she takes the bull by the horns, valiantly*): Mrs Keller, don't lose heart just because I'm not on my last legs. I have three big advantages over Dr Howe that money couldn't buy for you. One is his work behind me, I've read every word he wrote about it and he wasn't exactly what you'd call a man of few words. Another is to *be* young, why, I've got energy to do anything. The third is, I've been blind.† (*But it costs her something to say this.*)

KATE (*quietly*): Advantages.

ANNIE (*wry*): Well, some have the luck of the Irish, some do not.

KATE (*she smiles; she likes her*): What will you try to teach her first?

ANNIE: First, last, and – in between, language.

KATE: Language.

ANNIE: Language is to the mind more than light is to the eye. Dr Howe said that.

KATE: Language. (*She shakes her head.*) We can't get through to teach her to sit still. You *are* young, despite your years, to have such – confidence. Do you, inside?

ANNIE (*she studies her face; she likes her, too*): No, to tell you the truth I'm as shaky inside as a baby's rattle!

   (*They smile at each other, and* KATE *pats her hand.*)

KATE: Don't be. (JAMES *returns to usher them off.*) We'll do all we can to help, and to make you feel at home. Don't think of us as strangers, Miss Annie.

ANNIE (*cheerily*): Oh, strangers aren't so strange to me. I've known them all my life!

From *The Miracle Worker*, Act 1

* Dr Samuel Gridley Howe (1801–1876) was head of the Perkins Institution for the Blind in Boston. His tuition of Laura Bridgman, rendered blind and deaf by scarlet fever at the age of two, made him world famous. His reports on his cases were studied by Annie Sullivan before she accepted the position as teacher of Helen Keller when the latter became deaf and blind at the age of nineteen months.

† When Annie Sullivan was a young girl she was partially blind. She became a resident of the Perkins Institution four years after Dr Howe's death and was chosen by his successor as a person of exceptional talents who might be able to help Helen Keller. Helen's parents had applied to the Insitute for advice after her mother read Charles Dickens's account of his visit to Laura Bridgman in his *American Notes* (1842).

Sarah, deaf without speech from birth, but able to express herself fluently in sign language, passionately asserts her equal individuality as a human being and extols the virtues of Sign Language in Mark Medoff's play Children of a Lesser God.* *On the stage her speech is expressed in Sign Language and simultaneously read and spoken by James, a hearing speech teacher at a school for the deaf where Sarah is a student.*

SARAH and JAMES: For all my life I have been the creation of other people. The first thing I was ever able to understand was that everyone was supposed to hear but I couldn't and that was bad. Then they told me everyone was supposed to be smart but I was dumb. Then they said, oh no, I wasn't permanently dumb, only temporarily, but to be smart I had to become an imitation of the people who had from birth everything a person has to have to be good: ears that hear, eyes that read, brain that understands. Well, my brain understands a lot; and my eyes are my ears; and my hands are my voice; and my language, my speech, my ability to communicate is as great as yours. Greater, maybe, because I can communicate to you in one image an idea more complex than you can speak to each other in fifty words. For example, the sign 'to connect', a simple sign – but it means so much more when it is moved between us like this. Now it means to be joined in a shared relationship, to be individual yet as one. A whole concept just like that. Well, I want to be joined to other people, but for all my life people have spoken for me: *She* says; *she* means; *she* wants. As if there were no I. As if there were no-one in here who *could* understand. Until you let me be an individual, an *I*, just as you are, you will never truly be able to come inside my silence and know me. And until you can do that, I will never let myself know you. Until that time, we cannot be joined. We cannot share a relationship.

From *Children of a Lesser God*, Act 2

In his preface to the play Mark Medoff explains how it came to be written.

In January, 1977, I am in Rhode Island doing a workshop of a new play called *The Conversion of Aaron Weiss*. I have known the scenic and lighting designer Bob Steinberg for a year. He had done a lighting design for me a year before and is doing the set and lights for this production at the University of Rhode Island, where he is a member of the faculty. I am vaguely aware that, though a hearing person, he was in on the beginnings of the National Theatre for the Deaf; that he fell in love with one of NTD's actresses, Phyllis Frelich, deaf from birth. I know Phyllis 'retired' when they married and moved into the countryside of Rhode Island. I know they have two sons; Phyllis, they say, is busy being a mother and home-maker, but, boy, I should have seen her when she was an actress!

I am told that I will find Phyllis Frelich irresistible; everyone does. I prep myself to resist. *She's probably not that hot – deaf woman, handicapped, people feel sorry for her – overcompensate in praise. I won't fall for that.*

Our first 'conversation': I do not realize I am speaking loudly – as if she might hear if I get the decibel level up high enough. I also mouth my syllables carefully: *Hel-lo, Phyl-lis, I am so hap-py to meet you.* I am uninformed enough to think that all deaf people read lips. Many don't, Phyllis Frelich among them. (She comes from a family of eight deaf siblings, deaf parents. American Sign Language is their means of speaking; to them we're the ones who are handi-capped.)

I learn quickly that I don't know very damn much about deaf people. My experience runs to coughing up quarters in shopping centers for those little manual alphabet cards and somehow lump-ing the deaf all together with Patty Duke (a hearing actor) as Helen Keller in *The Miracle Worker*. Not exactly a comprehensive know-ledge of the subject.

Bob has to translate in order for Phyllis and me to talk. I immediately make another common mistake: I speak to *him* instead of her, as if she were in another country and he were some telephonic conduit. I am reminded of the cowboy and Indian movies of my childhood: *Tell Red Cloud me want be him friend.*

By the end of the second 'conversation' by which time I have

learned how to sign *How are you? I am fine* – not exactly 'com
munication' but I feel very frisky – I tell her I'll write a play for her

Why? Because she's a pitiable deaf lady? Because I want to 'save
the deaf and earn the undying gratitude of one of the last available
minorities? No. Because she points out to me that there are no parts
in the canon of 'hearing' theatre for deaf actors and because the two
of them – Phyllis *and* Bob – are separately and together . . . well
irresistible. Honest people, fiercely full of life and love, and as open
as any two people I've met.

They think it's a nice gesture – *He says he's going to write a play
for you* – but know it's just idle talk, the result of fascination
pleasant companionship, and a few drinks.

* The title of this play is often misunderstood. It is derived from
  Tennyson's 'Idylls of the King', which explains its true meaning:

> For why is all around us here
> As if some lesser god had made the world,
> But had not force to shape it as he would?

Verse

The Wife of Bath recounts how it came about that John, her fifth
husband, deafened her with a violent blow.*

What shall I say? Before the month was gone,
This gay young student, my delightful John,
Had married me in solemn festival.
I handed him the money, lands and all
That ever had been given me before;
This I repented later, more and more.
None of my pleasures would he let me seek.
By God, he smote me once upon the cheek
Because I tore a page out of his book,
And that's the reason why I am deaf. But look,
Stubborn I was, just like a lioness;
   Now let me tell you truly by St Thomas
About that book and why I tore the page
And how he smote me deaf in very rage . . .
   Who could imagine, who could figure out
The torture in my heart? It reached the top
And when I saw that he would never stop
Reading this cursed book, all night no doubt,
I suddenly grabbed and tore three pages out
Where he was reading, at the very place,
And fisted such a buffet in his face
That backwards down into our fire he fell.
   Then like a maddened lion, with a yell
He started up and smote me on the head,
And down I fell upon the floor for dead.
   And when he saw how motionless I lay
He was aghast and would have fled away,
But in the end I started to come to.
'O have you murdered me, you robber, you,
To get my land?' I said. 'Was that the game?
Before I'm dead I'll kiss you all the same.'

He came up close and kneeling gently down
He said, 'My love, my dearest Alison,
So help me God, I never again will hit
You, love; and if I did, you asked for it.
Forgive me!' But for all he was so meek,
I up at once and smote him on the cheek
And said, 'Take that to level up the score!
Now let me die, I can't speak any more.'
We had a mort of trouble and heavy weather
But in the end we made it up together.

From *The Canterbury Tales*,
translated by Neville Coghill

---

* A worthy *woman* from beside *Bath* city
was with us, somewhat deaf, which was a pity. (From the 'Prologue')

*This poem by the partially deaf French poet, Joachim du Bellay, is
addressed to Pierre de Ronsard whom illness deafened in his late
eens. Already a promising soldier and diplomat, he realised that his
career was jeopardised and decided 'to transfer the office of his ears
to his eyes'. He became one of France's best-known poets.*

All that I have of good, that in myself I value
Is to be without shame and without pretence, like you;
To prove a good comrade, and to keep good faith,
And to be, dear Ronsard, like you, half deaf:
Half deaf! What a fortune! Would to God I had had
Enough good luck to be deaf as an egg.
I am not one of those whose inflated poetry
Will create a mastodon out of a small fly,
But without altering a white to a black colour,
Or pretending a happiness to hide a dolour,
I will say that to be deaf – for those who know
The difference between good and evil (they are few) –
Is not an evil, only seems to be so.

From 'Hymn To Deafness', translated by David Wright.

JONATHAN SWIFT 1667–1745

Swift first experienced the symptoms of an incurable disease of the inner ear, now known as Menière's disease, when he was twenty-three years old. This condition which caused intermittent deafness, giddiness and nausea plagued him for the rest of his life.

ON HIS OWN DEAFNESS

Deaf, giddy, helpless, left alone,
To all my Friends a Burthen grown,
No more I hear my Church's Bell,
Than if it rang out to my Knell:
At Thunder now no more I start
Than at the Rumbling of a Cart;
Nay, what's incredible, alack!
I hardly hear a Woman's Clack.

ALEXANDER POPE 1688–1744

ON A CERTAIN LADY AT COURT*

I know the thing that's most uncommon;
    (Envy be silent and attend!)
I know a Reasonable Woman,
    Handsome and witty, yet a Friend.

Not warp'd by Passion, aw'd by Rumour,
    Not grave thro' Pride, or gay thro' Folly,
An equal Mixture of good Humour,
    And sensible soft Melancholy.

'Has she no Faults then (Envy says) Sir?'
    Yes she has one, I must aver:
When all the World conspires to praise her,
    The Woman's deaf, and does not hear.

* The Countess of Suffolk, mistress of George II. She is also referred to in a letter from Pope to Jonathan Swift dated 14 September 1725: 'I can also help you to a lady who is as deaf, though not so old as yourself; you will be pleased with one another . . . though you do not hear one another . . . What you will most wonder at is, she is considerable at court, yet no party woman, and lives in court, yet would be easy, and make you easy.' Swift replied (29 September): 'The lady whom you describe to live at court, to be deaf and no party woman, I take to be mythology . . .'

The deafness of Sir Joshua Reynolds, who is the subject of Gold-smith's epitaph, is attributed to a severe cold which he caught at the age of twenty-nine while studying Raphael's paintings in Rome. He used an ear-trumpet for the rest of his life. His 'Self portrait as a Deaf Man' is reproduced on the jacket of this book.

Here Reynolds is laid and, to tell you my mind,
He has not left a better or wiser behind:
His pencil was striking, resistless and grand,
His manners were gentle, complying and bland;
Still born to improve us in every part,
His pencil our faces, his manners our heart;
To coxcombs averse, yet most civilly steering,
When they judged without skill he was still hard of hearing;
When they talked of their Raphaels, Corregios and stuff,
He shifted his trumpet and only took snuff.

From *Retaliation: A Poem. Including Epitaphs
on the Most Distinguished Wits of this Metropolis*

Almost at the root
Of that tall pine, the shadow of whose bare
And slender stem, while here I sit at eve,
Oft stretches toward me, like a long straight path
Traced faintly in the greensward; there, beneath
A plain blue stone, a gentle Dalesman lies,
From whom, in early childhood, was withdrawn
The precious gift of hearing. He grew up
From year to year in loneliness of soul;
And this deep mountain-valley was to him
Soundless, with all its streams. The bird of dawn
Did never rouse this cottager from sleep
With startling summons; not for his delight
The vernal cuckoo shouted; not for him
Murmured the labouring bee. When stormy winds
Were working the broad bosom of the lake
Into a thousand, thousand sparkling waves,
Rocking the trees, or driving cloud on cloud
Along the sharp edge of yon lofty crags,
The agitated scene before his eye
Was silent as a picture: evermore
Were all things silent, wheresoe'er he moved; . . .

At length, when sixty years and five were told,
A slow disease insensibly consumed
The powers of nature; and a few short steps
Of friends and kindred bore him from his home
(Yon cottage shaded by the woody crags)
To the profounder stillness of the grave . . .
— And yon tall pine-tree, whose composing sound
Was wasted on the good man's living ear,
Hath now its own peculiar sanctity;
And, at the touch of every wandering breeze,
Murmurs, not idly, o'er his peaceful grave.

From *The Excursion*, Book 7

213

A TALE OF A TRUMPET

'Old woman, old woman, will you go a-shearing?
Speak a little louder, for I'm very hard of hearing.'
                                        – Old Ballad

Of all old women hard of hearing
The deafest, sure, was Dame Eleanor Spearing!
        On her head, it is true,
        Two flaps there grew,
    That serv'd for a pair of gold rings to go through,
But for any purpose of ears in a parley,
They heard no more than ears of barley.

    . . .

Deaf to sounds, as a ship out of soundings,
Deaf to verbs, and all their compoundings,
Adjective, noun, and adverb, and particle,
Deaf to even the definite article—
No verbal message was worth a pin,
Though you hired an earwig to carry it in!

    . . .

And yet the almond-oil she had tried,
And fifty infallible things beside,
Hot, and cold, and thick, and thin,
Dabb'd, and dribbled, and squirted in:
But all remedies fail'd; and though some it was clear
        (Like the brandy and salt
        We now exalt)
Had made a noise in the public ear,
She was just as deaf as ever, poor dear!

At last – one very fine day in June –
    Suppose her sitting,
    Busily knitting,
And humming she didn't quite know what tune;
    For nothing she heard but a sort of a whizz

. . .

However, except that ghost of a sound,
She sat in silence most profound—
The cat was purring about the mat,
But her Mistress heard no more of that
Than if it had been a boatswain's cat:
And as for the clock the moments nicking,
The Dame only gave it credit for ticking.
The bark of her dog she did not catch;
Nor yet the click of the lifted latch;
Nor yet the creak of the opening door;
Nor yet the fall of a foot on the floor –
But she saw the shadow that crept on her gown
And turned its skirt of a darker brown.

And lo! a man! – a pedlar! ay, marry,
With the little back-shop that such tradesmen carry,
Stock'd with brooches, ribbons and rings,
Spectacles, razors, and other odd things,
For lad and lass, as Autolycus sings

. . .

However, in the stranger came,
And, the moment he met the eyes of the Dame,
Threw her as knowing a nod as though
He had known her fifty long years ago;
And presto! before she could utter 'Jack' –
Much less 'Robinson' – open'd his pack –
    And then from amongst his portable gear,
With even more than a pedlar's tact,
(Slick himself might have envied the act) –
Before she had time to be deaf, in fact –
    Popp'd a trumpet into her ear.

'There ma'am! try it!
You needn't buy it –
The last New Patent – and nothing comes nigh it
For affording the Deaf, at little expense,
The sense of hearing, and hearing of sense!
A Real Blessing – and no mistake,
Invented for poor Humanity's sake;
For what can be a greater privation
Than playing dummy to all creation,
And only looking at conversation –
Great Philosophers talking like Platos,
And Members of Parliament moral as Catos,
And your ears as dull as waxy potatoes!
Not to name the mischievous quizzers,
Sharp as knives, but double as scissors,
Who get you to answer quite by guess
Yes for No, and No for Yes.'
('That's very true,' says Dame Eleanor S.)

. . .

'Try it – buy it – say ten and six –
The lowest price a miser could fix!
I don't pretend with horns of mine,
Like some in the advertising line,
To *magnify sounds* on such marvellous scales,
That the Sounds of a Cod seem as big as a Whale's;
But popular rumours, right or wrong,
Charity Sermons, short or long –
Lecture, Speech, Concerto, or Song,
All noises and voices, feeble and strong,
From the hum of a gnat to the clash of a gong,
This tube will deliver distinct and clear;
        Or supposing by chance
        You wish to dance,
Why it's putting a *Horn-pipe* into your ear!

216

          'Try it – buy it!
          Buy it – try it!
The last New Patent, and nothing comes nigh it,
          For guiding sounds to their proper tunnel!
Only try till the end of June,
And if you and the Trumpet are out of tune
          I'll turn it gratis into a Funnel!'

In short, the Pedlar so beset her, –
Lord Bacon couldn't have gammon'd her better, –
With flatteries plump and indirect,
And plied his tongue with such effect,
A tongue that could almost have butter'd a crumpet, –
The Deaf Old Woman bought the Trumpet.*

This long narrative poem is in three parts. Only the first part is
reproduced, much abridged by the editor. In the remainder of the
poem, Dame Eleanor, now able to hear due to her trumpet, turns into
a mischievous gossip and trouble-maker. She is finally drowned as a
witch by the angry villagers, aided by the pedlar. The poem ends
with a 'MORAL':

There are folks about Town – to name no names –
Who much resemble that deafest of Dames;
And over their tea, and muffins, and crumpets,
Circulate many a scandalous word,
And whisper tales they could only have heard
Through some such Diabolical Trumpets.

The subjects of the sculpture by Thomas Woolner, which inspired this poem, were Sir Arthur Fairbairn and his sister. Both were born deaf and without speech. Sir Arthur became a respected connoisseur philanthropist and champion of the profoundly deaf.

DEAF AND DUMB

A Group by Woolner

Only the prism's obstruction shows aright
The secret of a sunbeam, breaks its light
Into the jewelled bow from blankest white;
   So may a glory from defect arise:
Only by Deafness may the vexed Love wreak
Its insuppressive sense on brow and cheek,
Only by Dumbness adequately speak
   As favoured mouth could never, through the eyes.

The Walrus and the Carpenter on their nocturnal outing with lots of little oysters.

'But, wait a bit,' the Oysters cried,
    'Before we have our chat;
For some of us are out of breath,
    And all of us are fat!'
'No hurry!' said the Carpenter.
    They thanked him much for that.

'A loaf of bread,' the Walrus said,
    'Is what we chiefly need:
Pepper and vinegar besides
    Are very good indeed—
Now, if you're ready, Oysters dear,
    We can begin to feed.'

'But not on us!' the Oysters cried,
    Turning a little blue.
'After such a kindness, that would be
    A dismal thing to do!'
'The night is fine,' the Walrus said.
    'Do you admire the view?'

'It was so kind of you to come!
    And you are very nice!'
The Carpenter said nothing but
    'Cut us another slice:
I wish you were not quite so deaf—
    I've had to ask you twice!'

From *Through the Looking-Glass and What Alice Found There*

219

Heinrich von Treitschke, the German writer and historian, was deafened by illness as a child. He recounts the impact the experience had on him in a long poem written in rhyming couplets. It is offered here abridged in a prose translation.

A SICK MAN'S DREAMS

What a blessing is the cold winter breeze! How keenly and roughly it blows upon my cheeks! Never before have I greeted so joyfully the faint perfume of the first flowers to appear after the melting of the snow. I let you in through the window, a welcome guest, I drink in your fragrance with thirsty mouth. You bring me the first breath of life after I have lain so long in my bed, hot with fever. – Shut the window! My chest is still too weak. I will lie quietly here, look out on the broad expanse of sky, and once again, pleasure mixed with pain, cast my mind back to times long past.

In my mind's eye I can see my bedroom, so familiar and so dear to me, the scene of my noisy, boyish battles! Rays of light play upon the yellow wall while I, a sick child, lie in my narrow little bed. The small table has been pushed into a corner; my toy sabre, my constant companion, lies idle, no longer clinking at my side; my wooden horse, so long deserted, looks around for its rider with staring, questioning eyes. My parents are standing with a man who is a stranger to me – I wish I knew what they were talking about so quietly. He looks at them gravely and shrugs his shoulders. My mother weeps as if her heart would break.

O God! The fever was a treacherous old crone! It was not enough for her to fill the boy's days with pain; what she craved was to carry off his fresh young body to icy death in her withered arms. Many a night long, she sat at my bedside, trying to bewitch the hapless child with her evil eye, but she soon realised that I was too well protected by my parents' love. She admitted defeat, and just as she withdrew, full of rancour, she gave me a last kiss as a spiteful parting gesture. Old witch! Your kiss cast a spell upon me and it will take a lifetime to break it!

My father came to my bedside and put his lips close to my ear – I can still hear the echo of his well-loved voice: 'You are well again, you will soon be running about happily in the fresh air!' I made my way out of doors. It was as if an ice-cold arm had been laid around my breast. The sun still shone down, clear and warm; the garden seat, on which I used to rest, was still there; so too was the tree, at whose foot I used to listen to the twittering of the nestlings in its tall branches. But why, today, should their sweet song be stilled? Can it be that all gaiety has vanished from the earth? The farm girls are busy just as usual in the meadow, but why are they no longer singing their cheerful songs? The world of summer is sunk in wintry sleep. But no, listen! Now I can hear something – but alas, each sound is soft and muffled, reaching me as if from afar, unrecognisable, like a stranger's voice. Then I grew afraid. I raced back to the house, until my father called out to me: 'My poor son!' and told me of the malicious trick the fever had played on me . . .

And now I hear once again gentle and soothing sounds, echoes of long forgotten joys, like a greeting from fairyland. A word – a pressure of a hand – a loving kiss – and then the vision is lost in darkness. True, they were no more than words, short and trivial – you would laugh if I told you what they were – but the tones of that beloved voice were to me like the sound of a sea of joy. I would not take a kingdom in exchange for them!

Strange, magical word! What is a sound? Breath of a breath, the interaction of vibrating currents of air – listen! No sooner is it heard than it takes flight and is gone, lost in empty nothingness. Yet it possesses magical powers: it breathes life into the baby's cot; it unites whole nations in easy bondage – and where it is silent the abode of death is to be found . . .

The sounds which reach my ear mean less and less to me, the silence around me becomes ever deeper, ever more desolate; with the loss of hearing, I lose all zest for life, my friends have deserted me . . . Once again I am back in the hospital ward. Over there lie cripples with twisted bodies, and old, disabled men who are waiting for the doctor. Ah, life and all that fills it is sweet; no wonder that they want to put off their last journey as long as possible. Here I stand, tall, robust, and clear-eyed, a vigorous youth among all these aged men, and yet my affliction limps after me unseen, a derisive fellow-traveller, dogging my footsteps. Then

221

false shame and mortification overcame me. The bitter grief against which I have struggled so long grew to gigantic proportions and cursed and blasphemed my God, calling out to Him: 'Why didst Thou not strike me down with one of Thy thunderbolts? Thou art after all, well provided with terrors. How cruel Thou art! Must forever endure this unremitting torment, like a slave his fetters?' . . .

And what if the most dreadful of my fears should be realised What if such force of mind as remains to me should flag and wither away under the spell of cruel time? What if you should stand there helplessly, deaf and wretched? What if you should then brood in solitude, old before your time, stamp angrily and noisily upon the ground, and, like some madman, utter harsh screams and take childish delight in the sounds you have made? Will you then perish and find peace at last, a beggar and an outcast in the realm of sound? – No! I will stand firm in this bitter conflict. Life is too beautiful to be lost without a struggle . . .

No! You will hear what it is not given to everybody to hear, the most secret sounds within the human heart. You will be able to understand the reason for a troubled gaze and the cause of the deep blush which mantles a beautiful face. You will be second to none in what you can achieve: it is your task to sing the praise of courage that most powerful of consolations. Your words will give renewed strength to the sick hearts of those who patiently endure suffering and who do battle with the powers of darkness. Bright eyes can turn night into day and there is no affliction which does not bear within itself its own solace. Joy will accompany every step you take – how radiant it is! – and all your grief will prove to be no more than an illusion!

From *Krankentraüme*, translated by C. P. Magill

*The first book devoted to Corbière refers to his having become deaf
for a period of months. No medical documentation has
come to light.*

The specialist said: 'Let's leave it at that, couldn't be better.
The treatment's completed: you're deaf. The fact of the matter
Is you've completely lost the faculty.'
And not having heard, he understood perfectly.

—'Well, thank you sir, for having condescended
   To make a fine coffin of my head.
From now on, I'll be able to understand everything
   On trust, with legitimate vaunting . . .

Like window-shopping – But beware the jealous eye, in the place
Of the nailed-up ear! . . . – No – Why bother to defy?
. . . If in the face of ridicule I've whistled too high,
Below the belt it will sling mud in my face! . . .

I'm a dumb puppet, on a trite string!—
Tomorrow, a friend could take my hand, along the avenue,
Calling me: a bloody post . . . , or more kindly, nothing;
And I would answer 'Not bad, thanks, and you!'

If someone trumpets me a word, I go mad to understand;
If another is silent: would that be through pity? . . .
Always, like a *rebus*, I work to land
One word askew . . . – No. – So they've forgotten me!

—Or – the reverse of the coin – some officious being
Whose blubber lip makes the motion of grazing,
Believes he's conversing . . . While in torment
I put on an imbecile smile – with an air of discernment!

From 'Deaf Man's Rhapsody', translated by Val Warner

223

The explosion of George's 'Immense BALLOON'
causes a catastrophe.

When help arrived, among the dead
Were Cousin Mary, Little Fred,
The Footmen (both of them);
The Groom, the man that cleaned the Billiard-Room,
The Chaplain, and the Still-Room maid.
And I am dreadfully afraid
That Monsieur Champignon, the Chef,
Will now be permanently deaf –
And both his Aides are much the same;
While George, who was in part to blame,
Received, you will regret to hear,
A nasty lump behind the ear.

MORAL
The moral is that little boys
Should not be given dangerous toys.

> From 'George, Who Played with a
> Dangerous Toy, and suffered a Catastrophe
> of considerable Dimensions'

The subject of this poem is the poet's father.

ON A PORTRAIT OF A DEAF MAN

The kind old face, the egg-shaped head,
   The tie, discreetly loud,
The loosely fitting shooting clothes,
   A closely fitting shroud.

He liked old City dining-rooms,
   Potatoes in their skin,
But now his mouth is wide to let
   The London clay come in.

He took me on long silent walks
   In country lanes when young,
He knew the name of ev'ry bird
   But not the song it sung.

And when he could not hear me speak
   He smiled and looked so wise
That now I do not like to think
   Of maggots in his eyes.

He liked the rain-washed Cornish air
   And smell of ploughed-up soil,
He liked the landscape big and bare
   And painted it in oil.

But least of all he liked the place
   Which hangs on Highgate Hill
Of soaked Carrara-covered earth
   For Londoners to fill.

He would have liked to say good-bye,
    Shake hands with many friends,
In Highgate now his finger-bones
    Stick through his finger-ends.

You, God, who treat him thus and thus,
    Say 'Save his soul and pray.'
You ask me to believe You and
    I only see decay.

In this excerpt from his autobiography in verse the poet reveals that he became estranged from his father for some years as a result of not joining the family business.

My dear deaf father, how I loved him then
Before the years of our estrangement came!
The long calm walks on twilit evenings
Through Highgate New Town to the cinema:
The expeditions by North London trains
To dim forgotten stations, wooden shacks
On oil-lit flimsy platforms among fields
As yet unbuilt-on, deep in Middlesex . . .
We'd stand in dark antique shops while he talked,
Holding his deaf-appliance to his ear,
Lifting the ugly mouthpiece with a smile
Towards the flattered shopman. Most of all
I think my father loved me when we went
In early-morning pipe-smoke on the tram
Down to the Angel, visiting the Works.
'Fourth generation – yes, this is the boy.'

From *Summoned By Bells*

ROBERT PANARA 1920–

Robert Panara, Professor of English and Drama at the National Technical Institute for the Deaf (NTID), New York, became totally deaf from spinal meningitis at the age of ten.

ON HIS DEAFNESS

My ears are deaf, and yet I seem to hear
Sweet Nature's music and the songs of Man,
For I have learned from Fancy's artisan
How written words can thrill the inner ear
Just as they move the heart, and so for me
They also seem to ring out loud and free.

In silent study, I have learned to tell
Each secret shade of meaning and to hear
A magic harmony, at once sincere,
That somehow notes the tinkle of a bell,
The cooing of a dove, the swish of leaves,
The rain-drop's pitter-patter on the eaves,
The lover's sigh, the thrumming of guitar
And, if I choose, the rustle of a star!

They say I am deaf
These folks who call me friend
They do not comprehend

They say I'm deaf
And look on me as queer
Because I cannot hear

They say I'm deaf
I, who hear all day
My throbbing heart at play
The song the sunset sings
The joy of pretty things
The smile that greets my eye
Two lovers passing by
A brook, a tree, a bird,
Who says I haven't heard?

Aye, tho' it might seem odd
At night I oft hear God
So many kinds I get
Of happy songs and yet
They say I'm deaf.

In whatever condition, whole, blind, dumb,
Onelegged or leprous, the human being is,
I affirm the human condition is the same,
The heart half broken in ashes and in lies,
But sustained by the immensity of the divine.

Thus I too must praise out of a quiet ear
The great creation to which I owe I am
My grief and my love. O hear me if I cry
Among the din of birds deaf to their acclaim
Involved like them in the not unhearing air.

From 'Monologue of a Deaf Man'

THE FIFTH SENSE

A 65-year-old Cypriot Greek shepherd, Nicolis Loizou, was wounded by security forces early to-day. He was challenged twice; when he failed to answer, troops opened fire. A subsequent hospital examination showed that the man was deaf.

NEWS ITEM December 30, 1957

Lamps burn all the night
Here, where people must be watched and seen,
And I, a shepherd, Nicolis Loizou,
Wish for the dark, for I have been
Sure-footed in the dark, but now my sight
Stumbles amongst these beds, scattered white boulders,
As I lean towards my far slumbering house
With the night lying upon my shoulders.

My sight was always good,
Better than others. I could taste wine and bread
And name the field they spattered when the harvest
Broke. I could coil in the red
Scent of the fox out of a maze of wood
And grass. I could touch mist, I could touch breath.
But of my sharp senses I had only four.
The fifth one pinned me to my death.

The soldiers must have called
The word they needed: Halt. Not hearing it,
I was their failure, relaxed against the winter
Sky, the flag of their defeat.
With their five senses they could not have told
That I lacked one, and so they had to shoot.
They would fire at a rainbow if it had
A colour less than they were taught.

Christ said that when one sheep
Was lost, the rest meant nothing any more.
Here in this hospital, where others' breathing
Swings like a lantern in the polished floor
And squeezes those who cannot sleep,
I see how precious each thing is, how dear,
For I may never touch, smell, taste or see
Again, because I could not hear.

Called to the jury box, a prospective juror
asked to be excused because he was deaf
in one ear. 'No,' said the judge, 'that's no
impediment. You only have to hear one
side at a time.'

Contributed by Sir James Comyn

DEAF SCHOOL

The deaf children were monkey-nimble, fish-tremulous and
    sudden.
Their faces were alert and simple
Like faces of little animals, small night lemurs caught in the
    flash-light.
They lacked a dimension,
They lacked a subtle wavering aura of sound and responses to
    sound.
The whole body was removed
From the vibration of air, they lived through the eyes,
The clear simple look, the instant full attention.
Their selves were not woven into a voice
Which was woven into a face
Hearing itself, its own public and audience,
An apparition in camouflage, an assertion in doubt—
Their selves were hidden, and their faces looked out of hiding.
What they spoke with was a machine,
A manipulation of fingers, a control-panel of gestures
Out there in the alien space
Separated from them —

Their unused faces were simple lenses of watchfulness
Simple pools of earnest watchfulness

Their bodies were like their hands
Nimbler than bodies, like the hammers of a piano,
A puppet agility, a simple mechanical action
A blankness of hieroglyph
A stylised lettering
Spelling out approximate signals
While the self looked through, out of the face of simple
    concealment

A face not merely deaf, a face in darkness, a face unaware,
A face that was simply the front skin of the self concealed and
   separate.

Ted Hughes writes in a letter to the editor:

The piece of mine titled 'Deaf School' was really nothing more than a note, at the time, but I kept it just so because I did not feel I could do anything to it that would not blur the immediacy of the thing – which is its point.

When I worked in Paris with Peter Brook's Research Theatre in 1971 (I think), we were trying to find ways of dramatising certain things, effectively, *without language*. It was part of Peter Brook's long search for a Universal form of drama – a dramatic style, of acting, that would communicate at a deep level, clearly and powerfully, in spite of all language differences, class or cultural differences etc. Several times, in Paris, we – Peter Brook, the actors, and myself – visited a certain deaf school, where the actors and the children (around nine to eleven, as I remember) made little improvised plays together. I found these moving and fascinating. (I think we all did.) My piece was, as I say, simply a note made after one of these visits . . .

We found the deaf children incredibly quick and subtle in their perceptions, and expressive responses; wonderfully resourceful and – somehow – free, unself-conscious. They were certainly more inward and concentrated than non-deaf children of the same age – or they seemed so . . .

A song from the rock opera Tommy, *later made into a film by Ken Russell.*

Ever since I was a young boy I've played the silver ball;
From Soho down to Brighton, I must have played them all;
But I ain't seen nothin' like him In any amusement hall,
That deaf, dumb and blind kid sure plays a mean pin-ball.

Stands like a statue Becomes part of the machine
Feelin' all the bumpers, Always playin' clean;
He plays by intuition, The digit counters fall,
That deaf, dumb and blind kid sure plays a mean pin-ball . . .

Ain't got no distractions, Can't hear those buzzes and bells,
Don't see lights a-flashin' He plays by sense of smell.
Always has a replay, Never tilts at all,
That deaf, dumb and blind kid sure plays a mean pin-ball.
. . .

Even on my usual table, He can beat my best, –
His disciples lead him in, And he just does the rest.
He's got crazy flippin' fingers, never seen him fall,
That deaf, dumb and blind kid sure plays a mean pin-ball.

From 'Pinball Wizard'

234

TONY WONG 1951–

Tony Wong, a Jamaican, became paraplegic following an accident in 1978. He has been active ever since internationally on behalf of disabled people.

WHO IS DISABLED?

If you fail to see
the person
but only the disability,
then, who is blind?

If you cannot hear
your brother's
cry for justice,
who is deaf?

If you do not communicate with
your sister
but separate her from you,
who is disabled?

If your heart and your mind
do not reach out to
your neighbour,
who has the mental handicap?

If you do not stand up
for the rights of all
persons,
who is the cripple?

Your attitude towards
persons
with disabilities
may be our biggest handicap,
And yours too.

The Bible

And Moses said unto the LORD, 'O my Lord, I am not eloquent, neither heretofore, nor since thou has spoken unto thy servant: but I am slow of speech, and of a slow tongue.' And the LORD said unto him, 'Who hath made man's mouth? or who maketh the dumb, or deaf, or the seeing, or the blind? Have not I the LORD? Now therefore go, and I will be thy mouth, and teach thee what thou shalt say.

From Exodus, chapter 4

And the LORD spake unto Moses, saying, 'Speak unto all the congregation of the children of Israel, and say unto them . . . Thou shalt not curse the deaf, nor put a stumbling-block before the blind, but shalt fear thy God: I am the LORD.'

From Leviticus, chapter 19

Strengthen ye the weak hands,
And confirm the feeble knees.
Say to them that are of a fearful heart,
'Be strong, fear not:
Behold, your God will come with vengeance,
Even God with a recompense;
He will come anc save you.'
Then the eyes of the blind shall be opened,
And the ears of the deaf shall be unstopped.
Then shall the lame man leap as an hart,
And the tongue of the dumb sing . . .

From Isaiah, chapter 35

And again, departing from the coasts of Tyre and Siddon, he came unto the sea of Galilee, through the midst of the coasts of Decapolis. And they bring unto him one that was deaf, and had an impediment in his speech; and they beseech him to put his hand upon him. And he took him aside from the multitude, and put his fingers into his ears, and he spit, and touched his tongue; and looking up to heaven, he sighed, and saith unto him, 'EPHPHATA,' that is, 'Be opened.' And straightaway his ears were opened, and the string of his tongue was loosed, and he spake plain. And he charged them that they should tell no man: but the more he charged them, so much the more a great deal they published it; and were beyond measure astonished, saying, 'He hath done all things well: he maketh both the deaf to hear, and the dumb to speak.'

From Mark, chapter 7

Acknowledgements

The compiler gratefully acknowledges the publishers and authors below for their permission to reproduce, without fee, the following excerpts and poems:

Verily Anderson: from *Friends and Relations* (1980). Copyright © Verily Anderson 1980. Reprinted by permission of Hodder & Stoughton Ltd.

Prudence Andrew: from *Ordeal by Silence* (1961). Reprinted by permission of Century Hutchinson Ltd.

Jack Ashley: from *Journey into Silence* (1973). Reprinted by permission of The Bodley Head. Also from 'A Personal Account', in *Adjustment to Adult Hearing Loss* (Taylor & Francis, 1985). Reprinted by permission of the author.

Elizabeth Ayrton: from *The Cretan* (1963). Copyright © Elizabeth Ayrton 1963. Reprinted by permission of Hodder & Stoughton Ltd and of the author.

Patricia Beer: 'The Fifth Sense', from *Loss of the Magyar* (Longmans, Green, 1958). Reprinted by permission of the author.

Ludwig van Beethoven: 'Heiligenstadt Testament', from *The Letters of Beethoven* (1961), translated by Emily Anderson. Copyright © Emily Anderson 1961. Reprinted by permission of the Macmillan Press Ltd.

Brendan Behan: from *Borstal Boy* (1958). Copyright © Brendan Behan 1958. Reprinted by permission of Century Hutchinson Ltd.

Hilaire Belloc: from 'George, Who Played with a Dangerous Toy, and suffered a Catastrophe of considerable Dimensions', in *Cautionary Tales for Children* (1907). Reprinted by permission of Gerald Duckworth & Co. Ltd, and A. D. Peters & Co. Ltd, on behalf of the Estate of Hilaire Belloc.

Sir John Betjeman: 'On a Portrait of a Deaf Man', from *Collected Poems* (1958); and from *Summoned by Bells* (1960). Reprinted by permission of John Murray (Publishers) Ltd.

Elizabeth Bowen: from *Eva Trout* (Cape, 1969). Copyright © Elizabeth Bowen 1968. Also from 'Summer Night', in *The Collected Stories of Elizabeth Bowen* (1980). Reprinted by permission of Alfred A. Knopf, Inc.

Anita Brookner: from *Hotel du Lac* (Cape, 1984). Copyright © 1984 by Anita Brookner. Reprinted by permission of Pantheon Books, a division of Random House, Inc.

Geoffrey Chaucer: from *The Canterbury Tales*, translated by Neville Coghill (Penguin Classics, 1951, revised editions, 1958, 1960, 1975, 1977). Copyright © Neville Coghill 1951, copyright © the Estate of Neville Coghill 1958, 1960, 1970, 1977. Reprinted by permission of Penguin Books Ltd.

Carson McCullers: from *The Heart Is a Lonely Hunter* (Barrie & Jenkins, 1940). Copyright © 1940, 1967 by Carson McCullers. Reprinted by permission of Houghton Mifflin Company on behalf of the Estate of Carson McCullers.

Guy de Maupassant: from 'The Woodcocks' (also known as 'The Deaf-Mute'), in *The Complete Short Stories of Guy de Maupassant* (1970). Reprinted by permission of the Macmillan Publishing Co. Ltd., originally published by Cassell Ltd.

Mark Medoff: from *Children of a Lesser God* (1980). Copyright © Mark Medoff 1980, 1982. Reprinted by permission of William Morris Agency (UK) Ltd on behalf of the author.

Dorothy Miles: from *Gestures* (Joyce Motion Picture Co., Calif., 1976). Reprinted by permission of the author.

Vladimir Nabokov: from *Lolita* (Weidenfeld & Nicolson, 1955). Reprinted by permission of Mme Vera Nabokov.

Joy Packer: from *Boomerang* (Eyre Methuen, 1972). Copyright © 1972 by Joy Packer. Reprinted by permission of Anthony Sheil Associates Ltd on behalf of the Estate of Joy Packer.

Robert Panara: 'On His Deafness' (1947). Reprinted by permission of the author.

Arnold H. Payne: from *King Silence* (1918). Reprinted by permission of Jarrolds Publishers (London) Ltd.

Mervyn Peake: from *Mr Pye* (Heinemann, 1953). Reprinted by permission of the executors of the Estate of Mervyn Peake.

J. B. Priestley: from *Let the People Sing* (Heinemann, 1930). Reprinted by permission of A. D. Peters & Co. Ltd on behalf of the Estate of J. B. Priestley.

Elizabeth Quinn and Michael Owen: from *Listen to Me – The Story of Elizabeth Quinn* (1984). Reprinted by permission of Michael Joseph Ltd.

Jessica Rees: from *Sing a Song of Silence* (1983). Reprinted by permission of the author and The Kensall Press.

Jean Rhys: letter to Peggy Kirkaldy from *Jean Rhys Letters 1931–1966* (Deutsch, 1984). Reprinted by permission of Anthony Sheil Associates Ltd.

Jo Rice: from *Robbie's Mob* (1971). Reprinted by permission of William Heinemann Ltd.

Veronica Robinson: from *David in Silence* (Deutsch, 1965). Reprinted by permission of the author.

A. L. Rowse: from *A Cornish Childhood* (Cape, 1942). Reprinted by permission of the Crown Publishing Group on behalf of Clarkson N. Potter, Inc.

Tom Sharpe: from *Porterhouse Blue* (1974). Reprinted by permission of Secker & Warburg Ltd and of the author.

Edward Short (Lord Glenamara): from *I Knew My Place* (Macdonald, 1983). Reprinted by permission of the author.

Martin Cruz Smith: from *Gorky Park* (1981). Reprinted by permission of Knox Burger Assoc. Ltd.

Vian Smith: from *Martin Rides the Moor* (Longman Young Books, 1964). Copyright © Vian Smith 1964. Reprinted by permission of Doubleday & Company, Inc.

INDEX

The Quiet Ear is a rich anthology of pieces by and about the deaf which, Margaret Drabble says in her Preface, "quickens the senses of the reader and gives speech to a silent world." Anthologist Brian Grant, whose hearing was impaired by a war injury, has collected letters, anecdotes, fiction, poetry, drama and children's literature by writers from Mark Twain to Pete Townshend, Jane Austen to Carson McCullers. The selections are as varied as the authors in approach, ranging from serious to melodramatic to wildly comic.

To those who are deaf or partially deaf, *The Quiet Ear* will be as interesting for the misconceptions of the hearing authors as for the insights contained in autobiographical passages by Beethoven, Helen Keller and David Wright. To those who hear it will prove enlightening and revealing, and will surely influence attitudes toward the deaf.

"Out of very wide reading [Brian Grant has] compiled this collection of passages by and about deaf people, keeping a healthy balance between the comic and the melancholy, banal or tragic. . . . It is part of Brian Grant's humane mind and learning that he can both inform and amuse us at the same time."— *Birmingham Post*

"Here is an anthology from short passages of good writing. . . each illustrating some facet of daily living or thought by the deaf or some perception from the outside world about them. . . . The theme of deafness brings together unfamiliar passages from familiar writers. . . and, in attractive juxtaposition, fresh passages from the more obscure." — *Daily Telegraph*

"It is a volume everyone should dip into and a significant attempt to bridge the all-too-wide gulf that lies between the worlds of the deaf and those who can hear." — *Evening Chronicle*